GOLDBERG, Richard J. The psychosocial dimensions of cancer: a practical guide for health care providers, by Richard J. Goldberg and Robert M. Tull. Free Press, 1984 (c1983). 280p index 83-48069. 19.95 ISBN 0-02-911980-4. CIP

A well-written analysis of a variety of issues in the treatment of cancer. The authors first discuss children's comprehension of disease and death at various ages, and problems of young pediatric patients and their parents in relating to disease and treatment. Next examined are the special problems of adolescent patients, the psychological and social impacts of cancer on the adult patient, and support systems that mediate the impact of diagnosis and treatment. Chapters 4, 5, and 6 briefly review drug-related issues, and psychiatric symptoms having a physiological basis are analyzed with an extended discussion of depression and the use of antidepressants. Subsequent issues cover psychiatric symptoms of an iatrogenic nature, physical and psychological causes of nausea and vomiting in cancer patients, issues in pain control and the drugs used for this purpose, and the often unreasonable fear of "addiction." Psychosocial impact of the disease on the health professionals providing oncologic services is discussed, as is the use of the multidisciplinary team in oncology and the unique contributions of each team member. The final chapter explores the clinical and ethical problems inherent in issues of disclosure and refusal of treatment. Each of the chapters could be highly useful to health professionals treating cancer patients. Many should be read by a wider audience, including health profession students and families of cancer patients.—*L.A. Crandall, University of Florida*

The Psychosocial Dimensions of Cancer

A Practical Guide for Health Care Providers

Richard J. Goldberg, M.D.

Robert M. Tull, Ph.D.

THE FREE PRESS
A Division of Macmillan, Inc.
NEW YORK

Collier Macmillan Publishers
LONDON

The Free Press
A Division of Macmillan, Inc.
866 Third Avenue, New York, N.Y. 10022

Collier Macmillan Canada, Inc.

Printed in the United States of America

printing number
1   2   3   4   5   6   7   8   9   10

Library of Congress Cataloging in Publication Data

Goldberg, Richard J.
    The psychosocial dimensions of cancer.

    Includes index.
    1. Cancer—Psychological aspects. 2. Cancer—Social
aspects. I. Tull, Robert M. II. Title. [DNLM:
1. Neoplasms—Psychology. 2. Social environment.
QZ 200 G6194p]
RC262.G58   1983   362.1'96994   83-48069
ISBN 0-02-911980-4

OCLC

with appreciation to our families—
Sandra, Emily, Jenna, Karen, and Justin

Contents

Preface

MUCH OF THE MATERIAL in this book has come out of an extensive program in psychiatric oncology at Rhode Island Hospital. The foundations of this program were created in large part by Arvin Glicksman, M.D., Chief of Radiation Oncology and Andrew Slaby, M.D., Ph.D., Chief of Psychiatry. Their commitment to providing the highest standard of care and support for the integration of psychosocial dimension in medical care has fostered programmatic development in this area. Many others have contributed as members of the Psychiatry Oncology Program out of which this book developed, and we are grateful to the willingness of many disciplines to join us in an enterprise that intends to cut across discipline boundaries. Among those whose participation has been influential in the development of this book are Myron Boor, Bruno Borenstein, Denise Brown, Edwin Forman, Laura Hilderley, Stephanie LaFarge, Sharon Norman, Antoinette Pieroni, Norma Sullivan, Karen Weinstein, Margaret Wool, and William Worden. Beyond the substantial factual and clinical contents of the book, we hope it represents a concrete statement of a model that addresses the biologic, psychosocial, and existential dimensions of health care. Finally, we wish to thank the many providers and patients who shared personal experiences with us. We hope we have fulfilled their wish that we bring this material to the attention of other providers in this area.

Introduction

OVER THE PAST DECADE, advances in medical technologies have dramatically altered the experience of cancer. In the past, the diagnosis of cancer most often left the professional caregiver with the task of helping the patient prepare for death. Life extension and the cures now possible have created new challenges for everyone working with cancer patients and their families. With prolonged survival has come the need to pay more attention to the psychosocial dimensions of the cancer experience. New programs for patients, families, and staff have sprung into existence across the country, and there has been burgeoning interest in the fields of psychiatry, psychology, nursing, and social work in more focused work with oncology patients.

While the rewards of working in this field can be great, the challenges are often greater. Clinicians may remain at arm's length from their patients because of misconceptions and mythologies about the experience. The potential for intense emotional reactions can make them avoid the involvement with patients that can be so crucial to the treatment and rehabilitation process. Even for health care professionals, mistaken ideas about cancer are often forged from family mythologics or a few anecdotal experiences. Only recently have studies systematically assessed the psychosocial dimensions of the cancer experience. The first section of this book provides examples and discussion of a number of the key clinical issues encountered by those who work with children, adolescents, and adults with cancer.

Caregivers of all specialties must strive for an integration of the biomedical and psychosocial dimensions in the care of cancer patients. Too often, clinicians can jump to the conclusion that problematic emotional and behavioral responses are entirely accounted for by the psychological impact of having cancer. Commonly overlooked are changes in mood, thought, or behavior produced by the effects of the disease itself or its treatment. If identified, these organically based changes can often be reversed, thus restoring the patient's ability to cope with the situation. The second section of this book provides a detailed review of behavioral changes that are a physical consequence of the disease and many of its treatments. An additional chapter in this section devoted to issues of pain management will allow providers to become more knowledgeable and effective advocates in this area.

The final section of this book addresses issues related to caregivers and treatment programs. Many people who provide oncology care do so in relative isolation. Even when working as part of some larger organization, there is often not the opportunity to explore and metabolize some of the emotional impacts involved in this work. This section provides an opportunity to hear from other caregivers of various disciplines and can serve as a framework for exploring a number of common personal and ethical dimensions. If unattended, the problems can often lead to a decrease in professional satisfaction and efficacy. The needs of cancer patients and their families cannot always be met by single individuals. Increasingly, professionals of various backgrounds are simultaneously involved with a single patient, leading to potential confusion over roles and relations. We present parameters for a multidisciplinary mental health consultation team that clarify the unique and complementary roles of psychiatry, psychology, nursing, and social work in consultation to cancer patients.

This book is intended for professionals in all disciplines and their students who work with cancer patients. While caregivers from each profession may have specific tasks, they cannot isolate themselves from the patient as a whole person. Medical providers can become more effective by understanding the behavioral impact of their treatment as well as the psychosocial dimensions of the cancer experience. Social work, nursing, and psychology can become more effective by appreciating the interplay of biologic with psychosocial issues as well as by learning new therapeutic strategies or getting validation for current approaches. There have been a number of invaluable source books on issues involved in death and dying; this work is meant instead to provide practical information that will be immediately applicable to the clinical work of those involved with patients being treated for, and struggling to make sense of, their cancer experience.

PART I

Key Clinical Issues with Cancer Patients and Their Families

CHAPTER 1

The Child: Living with Cancer

INCREASINGLY, CHILDREN AFFLICTED with cancer are being cured of their disease. This is one of the great success stories of the past quarter century. Around 1950, acute leukemia, which accounts for at least half of childhood cancer, invariably was fatal within approximately three months after the onset of illness. By 1960, after the introduction of chemotherapy, some long-term survivors were already being identified. Now we can expect at least half of the children to be alive and well five years after the diagnosis of their illness. Many of these children have grown up and lead normal lives; some have married and have had children of their own. Similar successes have occurred in other forms of childhood cancer. Wilms' tumor, a cancer of the kidney that had an approximately 20% cure rate in the 1950s, is now cured in 80% of the children. Sarcoma of the soft tissue has an overall survival of 60% (Pinkel 1976; National Cancer Institute 1979, 1980).

The medical subspecialty, pediatric oncology, has recognized that children facing various life-threatening illnesses frequently encounter severe problems with psychological development and social interaction. As increasing numbers of children experience longer survival, new problems arise for patients and families (Koocher and O'Malley 1980). Questions include: What can be done to improve the quality of life for these children? How should life go on during treatment or in remission? How does the risk of relapse impair planning for and getting involved in the world?

With the success of cancer treatment in children, pediatric oncology services have had the opportunity to develop a model of optional care for patients. The model involves a variety of professionals knowledgeable in the issues crucial to helping the child withstand the tremendous interference of life-threatening illness and emerge as a functional adult. The historical medical model of care with an almost exclusive focus on biologic factors has been found inadequate because of the complex interaction of medical, psychological, ethical, and social issues that must be confronted in childhood cancer. Recognition of these multiple dimensions has led to the development of a philosophy regarding treatment, management, and psychosocial care that is more holistic and multidisciplinary in approach. Surgeons, radiologists, nurses, pathologists, chemotherapists, social workers, teachers, religious affiliates, dieticians, psychiatrists, and psychologists are facing the challenge to coordinate their disciplines with children and parents to assure integration to reach a common goal: the truly cured child (Van Eys 1977).* Recent research, although not conclusive, strongly suggests that the total psychosocial and familial setting, characterized by calm or by stress, has major effects on the response to treatment of disease (Dohrenwend and Dohrenwend 1974; Cobb 1974; Kaplan et al., 1977; Heller 1978; Caplan 1981). This chapter addresses a series of common issues and obstacles raised by the necessity of confronting cancer.

The Ill Child

How Does a Child Understand Serious Illness?

How a child reacts to hospitalization, chronic or life-threatening illness, treatment, and the threat of death depends greatly on the child's emotional-developmental age. It is important for staff and for parents, who are struggling to make sense out of a cascade of physical and emotional stresses, to try to put a child's internal experience in some context to guide their own behavior. As children develop and mature, their concept of life and death is a changing phenomenon. This evolving comprehension of serious illness generally can be categorized into various stages.

AGES 1 TO 5. The child from 1 to 5 years of age perceives death as a separation, as a state of being "less alive." It appears that the child does not quite recognize that death involves complete cessation of life, or that it is final (Nagy 1948; Anthony 1940). Children in this age range perceive the overall traumatic effect in terms of separation from their mothers, fathers, or the individuals who have given them the most nurturing since birth.

> Robert is a 3½-year-old boy with acute myelocytic leukemia who had relapsed three times over the previous year and was now having difficulty reattaining remission. The child had been presently hospitalized for over a month and was in the same room with another child, who was also at great risk of dying. For two nights, Robert had refused to sleep, and the staff had become increasingly concerned. When asked directly why he was not sleeping, the child could not come up with a response. When the staff psychologist suggested to the parents that they ask the child to draw a picture of what happened at night when the lights went out, he drew a picture, in dark colors, of the hospital room with two beds in it. In one bed was the sleeping roommate; the other bed was empty with a young child floating above it with a halo around his head. When the parents asked the child what the picture meant, the child explained that when he went to sleep at night, he died before his roommate did and he began to go up into the sky, but he wanted to wait so they could travel together and then return home next week.

This example illustrates three important points: the child defined death as a separation from his roommate; the child felt that death was transitory, and they would both return after a short period of "death"; and the child needed to express to his parents, through drawing, the fears that he was experiencing in the hospital. For young children, these might include fear of separation, fear of painful procedures, and fear of strangers.

Staff can encourage parents and older siblings to provide therapeutic interventions for a child of this age by encouraging the child's ability for creative expression in nonverbal forms. Drawing, clay, puppets, and various games are extremely valuable tools in helping children express and ventilate their feelings about having a serious illness. For example, in a group workshop (at Rhode Island Hospital) for siblings of cancer patients between the ages of 3 and 6, puppets are used to elicit the feelings that revolve around having a brother or sister with cancer. Children in the workshop create, draw, and cut out puppets of themselves and of their sick siblings who are being treated for cancer. The opportunity to express anger, jealousy, sadness, and caring is extremely important to the sibling who desperately needs a safe means of expression to help navigate through the crisis that has had such a major effect on the family.

For this young age group, it is really difficult to honestly approach the issue of death or of life-threatening illness. It is important, however, for the professionals and parents to listen carefully to what their child might be trying to express. When, for example, a young child is very sick, the parent must be as honest as possible in a way that the child can understand. From our extensive experience in pediatric oncology and from research that is presently emerging in the area, it is increasingly evident that children as young as 2 years old are aware of the impact of what is happening to them when they are facing a life-threatening illness. Most parents are extremely comforted to know that a child between the ages of two and five rarely asks directly, ''Am I going to die?'' But in the event that the child will ask, it is important that staff advise parents to address the question honestly yet gently. One parent explained to her 4-year-old child that he was very sick, and the doctors were doing everything they could to help her. In the final hours of her life, the child again asked if she were going to die. The mother, in a very moving gesture, embraced the child, held her tightly, and explained that whatever happened to her, she would be very safe, secure, and taken care of.

In other instances, the child will not bring up the issue of death directly, even when the parents have been extremely honest about the experience of treatment and the course of disease. In many cases, we found that children usually express a knowledge of what they are experiencing in nonverbal ways.

One 5-year-old boy with acute lymphocytic leukemia, who had been treated for four years, relapsed. He drew what he felt was going to happen to him. The mother, who was born in Brazil, wanted the child to be flown back home to be with her entire family at the time of his death. Extremely concerned about continuity of medical care, she took the risk of asking one of the pediatric oncologists if he would go with her and her family to South America to look after the boy in the final stages of his life. Although the mother had not expected the physician to say yes, he agreed, and the family, with the sick boy and the pediatric oncologist, prepared to travel to Brazil. About three days before they were ready to leave, the young boy, who had never asked his parents about what was going to happen to him or if he were going to die, drew a picture and handed it to them. The picture showed the little boy coming out of the water and on his way up into the sky. The water contained a big red monster, and the little boy was escaping it by going into the clouds. Over the little boy's head was the letter "J," representing the first initial of his name, John. It was clear to the boy's parents that this picture meant that John was aware that he was going to die and that he was going away from a very uncomfortable place into a safe haven in the sky.

It is apparent that children as young as 3 or 4 are extremely aware of the experience they are going through. Because the prognosis for cancer in this age group is extremely positive, it is even more important that parents understand their child's need to be dealt with honestly. It is our feeling that dealing with the issues directly with a young child whose prognosis and long-term survival are increasing will lead to less difficulty later on in life in terms of psychological adjustment to the world of being cured.

AGES 5 TO 9. Children between the ages of 5 and 9 begin to understand the finality of death. A child in this age group believes one might still be capable of eluding death; its inevitability and personal-reference components are not yet fully established. In addition, there remains a strong tendency to personify death (Spinetta 1981).

One 8-year-old girl, who had been treated for acute lymphocytic leukemia for 2½ years, had relapsed for the first time and was unable to reachieve remission. She was a bright child and still attended school when she was physically able. Her parents had been divorced for five years and the child lived with her mother, who provided almost exclusive, very supportive care to her and her 12-year-old brother. Approximately two days after being treated with a course of chemotherapy, she was playing in her room on the second floor of her home when the mother heard her scream. When her mother reached the foot of the stairs, the child was yelling that death was after her. She became so frightened that she jumped down the flight of stairs, crying hysterically and complaining that her hands were burning where death had tried to touch her. The mother packed her child into the car and rushed to the hospital; the child was trembling, flushed, and weepy. Although she was asked to explain her frightening experience, she refused to talk about it until the next afternoon. At that time, she was able to draw her perception of "The Death Man" and described in detail his attempt to capture her.

Rather than tell the child that her experience was just a bad dream, that would not happen again, it was important for her mother to acknowledge the experience and encourage her daughter to repeat in detail exactly what transpired. Through this process, the child was able to assume some control over her fear. She saw her mother remaining calm and was reassured that they would stick together in trying to elude this nightmare. The parent's response in sharing the experience in warding off bad thoughts plays an extremely valuable part in the parent's and child's ability to bond. These aversive "dreams" can even provide an opportunity for the parent and child to go through the illness in a much closer way.

Children between the ages of 5 and 9 begin to see death as inevitable and final. Despite the attempt of parents and staff to hide the seriousness of illness from children, recent research has shown that they understand the seriousness of their illness and experience fears of separation, bodily invasions, and abandonment (Spinetta et al. 1973, 1974).

AGE 9 AND UP.   From the age of approximately 9, children perceive death as both final and inevitable. Their concept of death undergoes a transition to that of an adolescent and adult.

One 10-year-old patient who had been treated for acute myelocytic leukemia was told by the oncologist that her disease was progressing, and they were having difficulty controlling the growth of the cancer cells. This 10-year-old previously had been an excellent skier and athlete, and the leukemia had resulted in medical complications that drastically limited her physical capabilities. Although this child never verbalized feelings about the disease, about a month before her death she wrote a beautiful piece of prose in her English class about running into a man selling baby blue balloons in the park. More than anything she had a great desire to buy a balloon, and after doing so the balloon burst—creating a huge pop, at which point she began to get smaller and smaller and rounder and rounder. She finally turned into a baby blue balloon herself, floating through the clouds and over buildings, and experiencing the most beautiful day in her life.

This example illustrates how one child can perceive death as final and inevitable, and yet as a freeing, beautiful experience—a mature and spiritual vision.

Although a child's understanding of death does not always follow predictable developmental lines, the sequence seems to be somewhat typical. It appears some children develop more mature concepts of the meaning of life and death if they are hospitalized or if they have a life-threatening illness. Once again, it is important to recognize children understand more than adults may assume. Oftentimes, it is the parent who best understands and knows the child's abilities, limits, and expectations. The parent can use many creative ways in which to verify some of the concepts the child is ready, or is not ready, to deal with.

As mentioned earlier, children this young tend not to express themselves verbally as directly as adults do. Their means of communication is direct but quite different. The use of puppets, drawings, and play therapy provides ways in which the staff and parents can directly communicate and understand. Parents may be uncomfortable or unfamiliar with such methods and should be encouraged to ask someone on the pediatric oncology service for specific suggestions. The staff should explore these issues with parents. Parents may feel they are protecting their child from painful issues but in reality may also not wish to face it themselves.

The Impact of Altered Body Image

The child facing a life-threatening illness frequently also faces the reality that most functional life-style activities are at least temporarily, and sometimes permanently, discontinued because of three major sources of interference: changes in physical condition and abilities; changes in peer relationships; and changes in family systems. These changes must be identified and addressed because progress in living and psychological growth depend on the ability of the sick child and immediate family to engage in activities that provide them with continued satisfaction.

Physical changes within the child are often brought about either by disease or by its treatment. These changes can be as subtle as lowered energy level, or as dramatic as hair loss, amputation, or impaired stature. The impact of these changes must be viewed in terms of the importance of their effects on the life-style of the individual child. Disruptions in the process of physical development and its related effects on body image can profoundly affect the child's psychosocial adjustment. For example, a theory of ''sociobiological advantage'' suggests that the child whose body type resembles the ''ideal'' enjoys special advantages and opportunities because of the favorable image he/she projects. Advertising, magazines, movies, television, and hero worship of athletes all contribute to glorification of the ideal body and disparagement of the deviant (Schonfeld, 1963). Such societal expectations imply that there are major risks for the child who undergoes alteration in body image. Seriously ill children are particularly fearful about what is happening to their bodies. Any insult that disrupts biologic integrity is automatically perceived in a heightened and exaggerated manner. Hair loss represents a major disruption in image that must be faced by children receiving treatment for cancer. For example, a young patient in third grade being treated for leukemia was extremely embarrassed and depressed for weeks after her wig accidentally fell off while she was in the school cafeteria.

> One mother related how, over a period of time of experiencing multiple hair losses, her child never wore a wig but preferred his old baseball hat. When Mark was diagnosed at age 3 with acute lymphocytic leukemia, the mother explained to him that he was receiving treatments to make him feel better and that one of the side effects would be that his hair would fall out, although it would grow back in time. The mother said that it was much more difficult for her to go through the experience of the hair loss than it was for the child himself. She noticed that as long as he had his baseball hat on, he did not appear to mind the treatments. The child was enrolled in a nursery school at the age of 3, and both the teacher and mother felt that the other

children accepted the baldness without any difficulty. The second time Mark lost his hair was when he was 5 years old. Before he returned to school at this time, his mother expressed her concern to the teacher over the difficulty that Mark and his school friends might have when he came back to the classroom. The teacher reassured the mother that she would prepare the class for Mark's return. She sat down with the class and explained that Mark had a disease called leukemia, which required the use of some very strong medications, some of which made him lose his hair temporarily. She pointed out that although the hair falls out for a period of time, it grows back, and that basically Mark was the same person he was before he lost his hair. Mark's integration into school was reported as very easy because of the enlightened and open message the teacher had shared with the class before his return. One afternoon, however, Mark and his mother met his father for lunch in the cafeteria at his father's place of work. Mark, dressed in his baseball hat, again appeared very calm about being in public with his hair loss. However, while he was sitting at the table, he realized that the other adults in the cafeteria were staring at him. The mother described how the boy took off his hat, turned around to the people, and yelled, "Why is everybody staring at me?" At this point, they turned around, stopped staring, and went back to eating.

Hair loss at various ages means different things to different children. The overwhelming issue remains that very often it is more difficult for the parents than it is for the child to go through this experience. It is the parents' responsibility, however, to reassure the child over and over again that the hair loss is temporary, that the hair will come back stronger and healthier than previously, that we can look at it in a different way and comb it in a different way to make it more of exciting to look forward to. But most important, the child must constantly be reassured that he or she is okay, and is still the same person as before the hair loss.

The embarrassment associated with body image changes threatens to deprive some children with a life-threatening illness of the benefit of the normal social interaction with peers that is necessary for maturation. Negative attitudes toward physical disability may result in such unhappiness in the school environment that a child feels driven to quit school and retreat from other social activities.

A 16-year-old girl was diagnosed and treated for acute leukemia. Prior to her illness, she was a bright, very attractive girl, who had been involved in children's theater productions for a number of years. After her initial treatments, she often insisted on not returning to school. Her parents, unguided by professional staff and deeply frightened by their daughter's near death, hovered protectively, reinforced her isolation, and though well meaning, actually reinforced her semi-invalid, outcast status. Not until she was readmitted to the hospital six months later for further treatment was it found out she had never returned to school and had spent most of her time watching television at home. She was angry, hostile, depressed, and socially isolated.

It is now well recognized that a child's integration back into normal activity is extremely important to psychological health (Katz et al. 1977; Kirten and Liverman 1977; Cyphert 1973). Most pediatric oncologists, except in exceptional medical circumstances, encourage their patients to return to school and extracurricular activities. If a student stays out of school for a long period of time, the parents or teacher might question the student and investigate the reasons and circumstances for not returning to school after the major intensive treatments have been completed. Returning to school, for a child with a life-threatening illness, is not particularly easy. The child may have experienced some kind of serious physical disability, ranging from an amputation to hair loss. The community is generally not informed as to the implications of cancer, and the stigma of cancer carries with it many strange ideas, including that it is contagious, or that it is always a "death sentence." When students with cancer return to school, very often they become the center of attention. Sometimes the attention seems very positive—books are carried for them, coats are brought to them, teachers may give them exceptional grades on tests. Although such aid is well-meaning, it probably is not helpful since it is a reminder of the patient's separate status (American Cancer Society 1980). In any case, it is usually short-lived.

What one could call the reputation of cancer can also lead to blatantly negative reactions that result in isolation from various activities, and to nasty remarks. As one young patient put it, "I'm always different; I'm either braver than the rest, or I'm weirder than the rest. I can never be normal." It is the role of the staff in the hospital, the parents, and the school system to cooperate to help children integrate back into the classroom in an appropriate way. Some patients and families choose not to tell the school about what they have been through. Other families and patients feel it is valuable for the class to have a discussion, before the child returns to the class, in terms of what to expect and what not to expect. The important factor is, however, that communication among parents, child, staff, and the school be open, and that it help to provide for the needs of the patient in the most appropriate fashion.

At Rhode Island Hospital, a consultation program with patients' school systems has been implemented by developing ongoing relationships with teachers, counselors, and administrators. With the consent of parents, all new patients' schools are contacted, and the medical status of the child, including disease and treatments, explained. The primary purpose of this contact is to establish healthy transitions of patients back into the classroom. The contact also will discuss how the school can facilitate the child's resumption of intellectual and social activities necessary for normal growth and development. Follow-up calls from the psychosocial staff provide further communication and allow the school to have any questions pertinent to the child answered. This program also provides ongoing consultation as well as yearly workshops on the biopsychosocial aspects of pediatric oncology.

Self-Blame

The tragedy of major illness is sudden and unexpected. It poses a direct challenge to those who feel life should make sense. The quest to reconstruct some sense out of the apparent lack of meaning is an important task. Like the patient, parents find it intolerable to think of their child's illness as a chance or meaningless event, and so attempt to create an explanation appropriate to their frame of reference. While scientific concepts of etiology provoke an acceptable explanatory framework for certain people, less rational reactions are ubiquitous. It is especially common for parents to blame themselves in some way. In such instances, the guilt associated with self-blame appears to be less anxiety provoking than living in a world that lacks any suitable explanation for the disease. This self-blame, however, may cause the parents to overindulge their child as a compensation for feelings of some earlier neglect. Initially, the child may enjoy such constant, specialized treatment, and the parents may take solace in the fact that they are doing everything possible, and more. However, since excessive dependency and loss of control are major hazards for the cancer patient, such overprotection may actually augment the helplessness and deprive the child of some of the self-determination necessary for developmental maturation. The child should not be expected to point this out. Most children are sufficiently ambivalent about their dependency–independency conflict that during the stress of illness they collude in such excesses.

It is not uncommon to hear of a 7-year-old, who, two years after initial diagnosis, demands that the parents do not go out with friends on a Saturday night, or insists on sleeping in the parents' bed. It can be especially difficult for parents not to be oversolicitous since their child's illness may allow them (at least temporarily) to enjoy the reestablishment of the more direct nurturing roles that are relinquished reluctantly as the child normally develops and moves closer to adulthood. Of course, parents want to see their child in good health again, and may believe that, magically, nurturing the child as an infant again may be curative. These feelings are quite common and should be acknowledged. Once such feelings are recognized, parents may gently redirect themselves from reestablishing the state of excessive dependency that may remove any sense of control from the youth.

Many parents become so personally involved in the lives of their sick children that they themselves become a deterrent to necessary rehabilitation procedures.

An 11-year-old boy was told of a shoulder amputation planned for treatment of his osteogenic sarcoma. His father's first reaction was, "He'll never be a man; he's better off dead." When it was discussed with the boy, he accepted it without major difficulty, and five years later was in a rehabilitation training program with the electricians' union. The father was later able to gain strength from his son's determination.

In another instance, a psychiatric consultant was called because of the unmanageable behavior of a 14-year-old boy who was admitted to the hospital for his first chemotherapy treatment. Although an average student who also got into his share of trouble at school, his behavior in the hospital was uncharacteristically nasty, and his constant complaining was frustrating to the nursing staff. The boy was loath to talk with the consultant initially, but the key to this problem was discovered in an interview with the father. The father, a serious practitioner of the martial arts, had instructed the doctor and nurses never to tell his son anything directly. Since he felt he knew his boy better than anyone else, he felt he should sift through any news about his treatment and present whatever information he felt his son should have. Because of the intimidating personal quality of the father, no one had really challenged him on this position. Furthermore, since his coping style involved denial of any emotional concerns, he brushed aside initial attempts to talk to him about his excessive censorship of his son's treatment. In this case, the consultant got the father to agree to participate in joint meetings with the doctor and his son, so direct communication with the boy could take place. Following the first meeting, in which the boy was able to hear the painful though undistorted news of his treatment from the doctor, which led to many questions, his behavior markedly improved, and he became one of the unit's favorite patients.

In general, we ought to indicate to overprotective parents that we understand their concern, and attempt to teach them such skills as how to offer support in a hopeful and encouraging manner, to aid the therapeutic regime, and to assist the young to return to permissible degrees of independence, self-management, and self-control.

For example, one 6-year-old boy being treated with chemotherapy agents for osteogenic sarcoma was experiencing extreme difficulty with nausea and vomiting. The child's father, having to watch helplessly as the child was debilitated by the treatments, became extremely agitated and demanding of the nursing staff. Fortunately, the child's primary nurse was trained in relaxation techniques and instructed the father on teaching the child various ways to relax. Both father and child were soon capable of handling these difficult circumstances with a mastery approach and supportive teamwork.

Parents, as well as patients, deserve staff tolerance, understanding, and support in developing changing roles when they are threatened by a serious illness. Parent groups throughout the country have helped to establish these goals, to provide support and validation as competent parents, and to increase the knowledge base for coping with the seriously ill child at home.

It is not easy for staff to develop parent groups to increase the social support of a family facing cancer. Many hospitals, however, begin this process by developing relationships with one or two parents who appear to be active participants in their child's care and who express a desire to "do something." Through this one-to-one staff–parent relationship, other parents can be solicited to participate in a self-help group designed to increase a family's ability to put the isolating experience of having a child with cancer in perspective.

Expanding the Medical Model

The historical medical model that demands blind acceptance of a medically prescribed regimen, relinquishment of preillness duties and rights, and the adoption of deviant status reinforces the concept of the child as a passive recipient of external forces over which he/she has no direct control. Families as well often succumb to this dependent role and find responsibility for the sick child passing progressively out of their hands into those of specialized extrafamilial agencies.

It appears that an unfortunate, though common, pattern emerges when a child enters many pediatric units. The child generally needs someone to help him/her cope with the incredible stresses and novel environment encountered at onset of disease. It is at this point that the fragmentation begins. The doctors consider the biologic care so paramount that many tend to ignore, or sometimes even degrade, other concerns. The nurses, truly on the front lines of care, think of themselves as the primary person to support the child. The social and mental health services become advocates for programs in which health care is seen as only a minor part of the child's needs. The pastoral services consider the spirit paramount and seek to become the purveyors of health. As a result, the roles become duplicated and competitive (Van Eys 1977). In addition, all internal groups begin to feel threatened when others begin to scrutinize their specific roles. Where are the parents in all this? The parents are, after all, the long-standing social supports and caretakers of the child. They know the child better than any professional ever could through a brief basis. Not only do the professionals create a risk of confusion in their competition to care for the child, but in their enthusiasm they overlook the negative consequences of ''replacing'' the parents as the true caretakers. In most cases, the professionals should work to help the parents become more effective supports rather than to replace and bypass them.

The old model of care, where one physician attempted to be responsible for all treatment, is clearly inadequate to the needs of the pediatric oncology patient. The work of the physician must be supplemented and coordinated with professionals who provide for and attend to a variety of needs, including nursing, educational, psychological, and social (Koocher and Sallan 1978; Sheldon et al. 1970; Hoffman et al. 1976). (See chapter 9.) While there is no model yet universally agreed upon, there are currently a number of ongoing experiments in such team approaches in which participants, which include the parents and patient, relate more openly to each other and cooperatively think through management decisions for the child with cancer. However, we all must remember that the sick child is the center of the treatment team. It is the child who is receiving the drugs, undergoing the operation, receiving the radiation therapy. Therefore, parents and staff must make the greatest effort to explain, in an age-appropriate manner, the implications, treatments, and potential side effects that the child will experience. One of the major issues that faces a child with cancer is a sense of loss of control over the normal way of life. When the chemotherapist asks the child to sign a treatment consent form, after explaining some of the side effects, such a process recognizes the rights of children to know what they are going through. The surgeon approaches a 7-year-old girl, explains to her about her amputation for her osteogenic sarcoma, and asks her and her parents to sign a consent form, and thus the child's sense of control over her own illness is increased. It is the recognition of the child as a person which will alleviate some of the stress that goes along with the parents' sense of responsibility and the medical sense of responsibility. It places children in the position of being not only the patients but also members of the treatment team themselves.

This chapter has addressed four core issues that are basic for professionals attempting to deal effectively with chidren with cancer. First, there should be some understanding of the process of development of death awareness and how a child's stage of awareness guides management approaches. It is of paramount importance that each child be given stage-appropriate communication on subjects that can free the child's emotional energy from the struggle with the unknown. One must be sensitive to the child's needs for understanding, reassurance, and reaffirmation of hope.

A second area of key importance is the recognition of the intimate relationship between altered body image and self-concept. Unless this issue is recognized and addressed in some way, unnecessary social isolation and permanent psychosocial deficits may result. Third, the tendency of parents to blame themselves for the onset of cancer in their child is a predictable reaction that should be open to discussion to avert dysfunctional styles of parental caretaking. Finally, parents and professionals alike must recognize how traditional systems of care create iatrogenic fragmentation of the social support system that remains crucial to adaptation to illness and quality of life.

References

AMERICAN CANCER SOCIETY: *Parent's Handbook, Rhode Island Hospital* (1980).

ANTHONY, S.: *The child's discovery of death*. New York: Harcourt Brace, 1940.

CAPLAN, G.: Mastery of stress: psychological aspects. *Am. J. Psychiatry* 138 (Apr. 1981).

COBB, S.: A model for life events and their consequences. In B. S. Dohrenwend and B. Dohrenwend (Eds.), *Stressful life events*. New York: Wiley, 1974.

CYPHERT, FREDRICK, R.: Back to school for the child with cancer, *J. School Health* XL111 (Apr. 1973), 215–217.

DOHRENWEND, B. S., AND DOHRENWEND, B. (EDS.): *Stressful life events. Their nature and effects*. New York: Wiley, 1974.

HELLER, K.: The effects of social support: Prevention and treatment implications. In A. P. Goldstein and P. H. Kanfer (Eds.), *Maximizing treatment gains: transfer enhancement in psychotherapy*. New York: Academic Press, 1978.

HOFFMAN, A., BECKER, R. D., AND GABRIEL P. H.: *The hospitalized adolescent: A guide to managing the ill and injured youth*. New York: Free Press, 1976.

KAPLAN, R. H., CASSEL, J. C., AND GORE, S.: Social support and health. *Med. Care* 15 (1977), 5: 471–482, supplement.

KATZ, E., KELLERMAN, J., KIGLER, D., WILLIAMS, K. O., AND SIEGEL, S. E.: School intervention with pediatric cancer patients. *J. Pediatr. Psychol.*, 2: 72–76, 1977.

KIRTEN, D., AND LIVERMAN, M.: Special education needs of the child with cancer. *J. School Health* 170–173, 1977.

KOOCHER, G. P., AND O'MALLEY, J. E. (EDS.): *The Damocles syndrome: Psychosocial consequences of surviving childhood cancer.* New York: Mc-Graw-Hill, 1980.

KOOCHER, G. P., AND SALLAN, S. E.: Pediatric oncology. In P. Magrob (Ed.), *Psychological management of pediatric problems* Vol 1. *Early life conditions and chronic diseases.* Baltimore: University Park Press, 1978.

NAGY, MARIA: The child's theories concerning death. *J. Genet. Psychol.* 73 (1948): 3, 27.

NATIONAL CANCER INSTITUTE: *Coping with cancer: A resource for the health professional.* Bethesda: U.S. Department of Health and Human Services, 1979.

NATIONAL CANCER INSTITUTE: *Coping with cancer: A resource for the health professional.* Bethesda: U.S. Department of Health and Human Services, 1980.

PINKEL, DONALD: Curability of childhood cancer. *JAMA* 235 (Mar. 1976) (10): 1049–1050.

SCHONFELD, W. A.: Body image in adolescence: a psychiatric concept for the pediatrician. *Pediatrics* 31 (1963): 845.

SHELDON, ALAN, CHIR, B., RYSER, CAROL, AND KRANT, M.: An integrated family oriented cancer care program: The report of a pilot project in the socio-emotional management of chronic disease. *J. Chron. Dis.* 22 (Apr. 1970): 743–755.

SPINETTA, JOHN: Psychosocial issues in childhood cancer: How the professional can help. in Paul Ahmed (Ed.), *Living and dying with cancer.* New York: Elsevier, 1981, pp. 53–77.

SPINETTA, J.: The dying child's awareness of death: A review. *Psychol. Bull.*, 81 (1974): 256–260.

VAN EYS, J. (ED.): *The truly cured child: The new challenge in pediatric cancer care.* Baltimore: University Park Press, 1977.

CHAPTER 2

===

The Adolescent

CANCER REMAINS THE MOST common life-threatening illness for adolescents. Recent developments in cancer treatment have created a more encouraging and optimistic view of the course of the disease. In the 1950s, a young cancer patient was usually viewed as terminally ill. Medical and nursing care, therefore, centered around palliative treatment. Now, adolescents with cancer spend fewer days in the hospital and more days in their home, school, or work environment (Van Eys 1977).

The psychosocial problems to be faced with cancer are no longer limited to dealing with death and dying. As treatment methods have created more chronic forms of illness, new attention to rehabilitative issues become especially important. Getting on with life and growing up are now real concerns for many cancer patients who were formerly branded as exiles from the world. New scientific developments and increased cure rates have also led to special problems of living with cancer. Among the major concerns of the adolescent cancer patient is the uncertainty that pervades remission, creating hope as well as suspense and stress (Koocher and O'Mally 1973; Pfefferbaum and Levenson 1982).

One adolescent said:

> When they first told me I had leukemia, I automatically thought, how much longer do I have to live?
> They just said, "You have leukemia." They told me what it was and everything like that, and I had seen this movie on television about a kid who had leukemia and he died. Naturally, I thought that was going to happen to me. I thought it was the end of being on earth. I really wasn't crying so much for myself. It's just that everybody, like my dog, would miss me. My parents would miss me, and you know how they felt. They would probably feel that it was all their fault.

The psychological impact of cancer can be more devastating during adolescence than at other ages because of the additional stresses associated with achieving independence and consolidating identity. The growing pains that accompany emergence into adulthood typically felt by normal adolescents are acutely aggravated by the feelings of helplessness and loss of control imposed by the disease and aggressive long-range treatment modalities it involves. Neither the child, too young to understand the meaning of malignancy and without a clear concept of death, nor the adult, who has lived a long life and developed coping strategies for major life stresses, is burdened with these additional strains. The adolescent occupies a precarious and vulnerable position: mature enough to realize the implications of the diagnosis and prognosis but not equipped with the full range of coping mechanisms of the older adult. As seriously ill adolescents attempt to fulfill their developmental tasks, they face such serious conflicts as fear of the unknown surgical experiences or other bodily invasions, confusion and anxiety about the outcome of the illness, distress as a result of forced dependency, alterations in the body image, isolation from peers, diminished self-esteem, interference with educational and vocational plans, and impact upon hopes for marriage and family (Hoffman and Becker 1973).

Despite the incredible strains of growing up with cancer, adolescents with serious illness can avoid permanent psychological damage and perhaps even grow because of it. Many adolescents are able to develop coping strategies to overcome successfully the psychological challenges posed by their disease and that eventually lead them to become well-adjusted adults. Many people feel that because of their honest straightforwardness and confrontative personalities, adolescents may even have a better chance than adults in coping with cancer.

This chapter takes a closer look at the effects of illness and hospitalization on the normal developmental process of the adolescent and the predominant concerns of the adolescent cancer patient. Throughout the chapter, we quote from members of our adolescent groups of cancer patients who provide eloquent descriptions of their important issues.

Changes in Body Image

Body changes can be awkward and confusing for some, and for others a joyful triumph. For most adolescents, they are inevitable. This is not so for many cancer patients. Growth changes generally occur in all individuals, but the magnitude and times of onset and completion may be quite variable depending on genetic inheritance, sex, race, nutrition, previous illness, and environment. On the average, the growth spurt in boys occurs between 13 and 15½ years of age. In girls, this spurt begins at about 11½ years and is almost complete by 13½ years. Changes in the reproductive and endocrine systems lead to alterations in facial contours, fat distribution, pelvic proportions, and muscular development that bring the child toward adult stature (Tanner 1962). This development of body image is one of the major concerns of the adolescent and is closely interwoven with the individual's self-concept. Physical impairment constrains freedom of movement and self-determination as well as involvement in the supportive peer environment. The consolidation of gross motor skills, through athletics for example, helps the adolescent gain control over the environment. Emotional development depends a great deal on peer interaction, which in turn is dramatically influenced at this age by body image. Those who are excessively self-conscious or seen as physically "different" are at risk for exclusion from the socialization required to develop autonomy, academic and vocational options, and sexual identity. Through its pervasive and sometimes dramatic effects on body image, cancer has a potentially serious impact on many developmental areas (Kellerman and Katz 1977; Hoffman and Becker 1973). One adolescent commented,

I used to run cross country all the time. I wasn't that terrific at it, but I enjoyed it. Now when I run I lose my breath faster and everything, and get tired much quicker, so I gave that up and began to do something else that's not as strenuous, like swimming for ten minutes instead of an hour. You know, you can still do the things you like, except you have to watch the time limits on them.

Recognition of physical limitations as well as emotional capabilities must be frequently assessed for the young person facing a life-threatening illness. Parents and staff can assist in being supportive by suggesting various alternatives to their adolescent that are more in tune with their physical abilities. We have seen instances where high school track stars have become coaches, or where joggers have switched to the less strenuous bicycle. Parents also can realize that adolescents can determine independently what is right for them.

As one patient said:

I think a lot of the time it's the medication that I blame. You just can't keep up; you just run out of breath faster. You can't spend as much time doing things, but it's been this way for me for so long, I found I've developed my taste around that. I've had to substitute things, like swimming and running for badminton, Ping-Pong, and volleyball, things that don't require a lot of running, and I like to write. I think it's just like redefining the activities I've chosen.

Another commented:

I always have had a hard time accepting that I was limited in any way. In high school I was wrestling, and you just can't wrestle in moderation. I'd just go out and do things until I guess I dropped, and then I'd call home and tell my parents I couldn't do it anymore. They'd suggest other alternatives that were less strenuous.

And another stated:

I want to keep fighting this. I keep saying to myself, "Well, this winter I'm going to lift weights or something to build up my strength, so in the spring it'll be just like it always was." I just can't accept; I just can't give it up yet. I've always been a real fighter, so I'm gonna try to fight this all along. You don't want things to change that are good, that you enjoy. I still have a lot of hope, so I'll keep on trying.

Despite the diagnosis of cancer, it is important to the achievement of autonomy during adolescence for these young people to continue to develop increasingly greater levels of control over themselves and their environment (Erikson 1950). These quotes from a group of adolescent cancer patients are an example of the kinds of issues that the patient experiences with a life-threatening illness. Both the adolescent male and female are more vulnerable today because of the sex-role expectancies to become strong and masterful. Many acceptable activities are "action oriented" and involved in "doing." Consequently, conditions that interfere with action-oriented successes, especially in early and midadolescence, will be particularly stressful to patients who are not able to reorient their objectives and goals (Hoffman and Becker 1973).

As one girl said:

I remember when I had my wig. We were just starting trampolines. You can imagine that. I told my mom about it, and she said, "Well, we can get you a little rubber strap to put under your chin, and that will hold it on." That didn't turn me on at all. I would rather skip gym during that period than get on that trampoline and have my wig bounce off.

It is important for staff not to overprotect and smother patients, but to recognize the importance for the adolescent to continue activity in other acceptable ways.

Whereas visually evident handicaps can be measured in a clear and concise reality, conditions not so readily apparent are more difficult to assess and may cause confusion in self-perception and body image. For example, one 18-year-old young man said:

As far as keeping up with my friends, after 3½ years they understand, but at first they used to feel sorry for me. I was exhausted, and I just couldn't keep up with them. Now I just say, "Go ahead, and I'll catch up with you in a little while," or I'll just go home and take a nap. I guess at first they didn't understand because they didn't think that anything was wrong with me. The main thing now is that they understand, so it helps me because, when people don't know how you feel, they don't know how to treat you and be with you. It's better just to tell them right out. You just give them the truth, and often they say, "Oh, why didn't you tell me?" It's a totally different story after they know.

With leukemia you can't tell that you're sick. I mean, people look at you and say, "What's wrong?" When I was staying in a hospital, in third grade, when I relapsed, I had a roommate who asked me that very question. "Why are you here, you don't look sick?" "I have leukemia," I said. She hit the wall. "Is it contagious?" "No, you wouldn't be put here if it was contagious," I said. "Are you sure?" she said. People don't know how to react until they know what the score is.

The honesty and directness of the adolescent having cancer can be a valuable learning experience for parents and staff. One parent, after hearing her adolescent discuss the issues of how she dealt with her cancer, said, "I've learned so much from my daughter about the benefits of being honest and direct that it has helped my own personal growth."

Peer Group Membership

It was like I was a piece of glass. Nobody wanted to get near me. They were afraid I was going to break.

When you have leukemia or some kind of disease most people don't have, there are a lot of things like side effects and drugs, being tired, being sick, not having the energy other people have, having to go for treatments, having to deal with doctors and hospital situations that set you apart from your peers. I guess everybody feels alone, but it seems to me that there is much more that you don't have in common, and that can be lonely . . . When I was little, my one wish was to be normal, and I realize now that that was sort of silly because nobody knows what that is, but I guess that's something people try all their lives to accomplish.

Peer membership involves the development of friendships that help to bring about self-understanding and self-acceptance (Daniel 1970). Having a chance to verbalize feelings and ask questions is necessary for justifying beliefs and for clarifying concepts not previously existent. A strong friendship often serves to comfort hurts, lend courage, and provide reassurance that thoughts and actions are shared by someone else. Friends mean acceptance and increased self-esteem. Friendships during early adolescence are used more for support and mutual understanding while parents are still accepted as having decision-making roles and final authority. During later adolescence, the influence of peer groups assumes greater importance and can replace the views and standards set by parents. Concepts of independence and self-determination are accomplished through the individual social network. While an adolescent with cancer has significant problems with social and peer activity, it is important, despite the illness, that such relationships be maintained to promote self-esteem and diminish the fears of rejection and abandonment. Some patients are subject to cruel and unthoughtful remarks by peers. One young girl tells a story of how she went back to school, and one kid came up and said, "So, when's your time up? When're you gonna bite the dust?"

For parents, having to witness such thoughtless and cruel remarks might be one of the most difficult experiences involved with the illness. Their normal impulse is to protect the child, become angry, and confront the offender. Many parents say they never forget such incidents. The parent might ask; How do I deal with a situation like this? How do I help defend my child against thoughtless remarks and insensitive comments? One young girl who had just completed treatment for a brain tumor and was wearing a wig was having a difficult time with her peers at school. On numerous occasions, her schoolmates did not ask her to walk with them a mile and a half to a fast-food restaurant during lunch hour because they were afraid she would become too tired. As a result, the young girl felt her friends were angry with her, and she expressed this hurt to her mother. Her mother's immediate reaction was to call the other mothers, and to complain about the girls' unforgiveable behavior. The result at school was that the other girls were so put off by the mother's interference that they became even more distant and withdrawn. When someone finally disclosed what had transpired, the young patient was able to discuss the subject with her friends and they resolved the difficulty among themselves. Although the parent can feel the hurt of seeing normal social activity curtailed because of the illness, it is important to avoid intrusions into peer relationships. Instead, parents can explain that other teenagers may act cruelly because they feel threatened, because the notion of cancer confronts them with their own vulnerability to disease, weakness, and possible disfigurement. Parents can assure the patient that they know more about the hopeful nature of the disease than do the patient's peers. We are aware from extensive interviews that healthy teenagers are often groping for the right way to act, and it may be up to the patient and the parents to take some initiative in helping to reestablish these strained relationships:

> When you're having a hard time coping with everything, you find out who your friends really are. Before I was sick, I used to hang around these kids. Then I went into the hospital. Friends came to visit me, or they came over to see me at my house when I was sick. Some kids, however, you don't see unless you go over to them. So it really singles out who your best friends are. Once I ran into this kid that I hadn't seen since I've been sick, and we were just talking, and he said, "I never hung around with you because you have leukemia." I said, "Why?" He said, "Well, I was scared. I didn't want to say something that would hurt you or anything." So I just told him how good seeing him was and said, "You should talk about it; ask me questions, I don't care." Now we're a lot closer, and it was just because this kid was afraid to speak up that he never hung around me, but we have a lot of good times together now; it's very nice.
>
> Talking about it with friends is a lot better. You get things straightened out. It makes you feel less in isolation and just like everybody else, only you have a disease. It's not like you're from some other planet or something.

The importance of peer groups among patients is becoming increasingly clear. Such groups provide crucial socialization and activities that might otherwise be missed. Many hospitals are now developing such therapeutic programs for both hospitalized and outpatient adolescents. Some community agencies, such as the American Cancer Society, are also beginning to design programs for the adolescent patient. A framework in which adolescents can ventilate and work through their anxieties, reaffirm peer group acceptance through social and recreational interaction, and constructively assume independence and control through achievements in various activities programs can be very beneficial. The implementation of this kind of system depends upon the establishment of firm, interlocking lines of communication among staff, patient, and family groupings with a clear understanding and respect for the various roles of all involved. It is through the sensitive understanding of the pediatrician who maintains strong relationships with the psychosocial staff that successful patient, sibling, and parent groups can be organized. For the adolescent, who can feel very much alone and isolated and perceives others as hostile and uncaring, these programs can focus on the strengths and positive qualities, and, more important, give the adolescent meaning through warm, nonjudgmental contact, while helping to retain ties to the world and others. The strategy of group programs is to increase long-term adjustment for the patient through better interpersonal relationships.

Therapeutic Interventions

Approximately three years ago in the Department of Pediatric Oncology and the Department of Psychiatry at Rhode Island Hospital, it was found through various staff members that many of the adolescents being treated for cancer were experiencing a sense of wanting to meet others in similar circumstances. We also discovered that these adolescents were extremely interested in providing some service or in doing some meaningful task to help others going through a similar process. As an experiment, the two departments helped bring together a small group of adolescent patients, ranging in age from 13 to 20, to meet outside the hospital on neutral territory to discuss the emotional issues involved with cancer, and to develop ways to help educate the community, the caregivers, and new patients as to what it is like for a young person to experience cancer. The first group met with two staff psychologists for a period of six weeks. A videotape camera recorded the entire process at each session. Meals were generally served prior to the sessions to help generate relationships among the participants; in most instances, they had not known each other previously, except for occasional chance meetings in the clinic on treatment days.

As the sessions progressed, both the co-leaders and the group members began to realize that the material being taped was extremely valuable information that could help the community and the hospital staff better understand what the experience of cancer was like. However, some of the participants could not believe that what they were saying would be valuable information for physicians. Therefore, a joint taping was arranged with the oncologists to discuss how the doctors felt about the tapes and how the tapes helped them to do their jobs better. When all sessions were completed (about 20 hours of videotape), transcripts were made of the entire group sessions, and distributed to the participants. Each member was asked to edit all parts of the tape that needed to be worked on. The participants decided which pieces were valuable, and which pieces were not that important and should be deleted. Then, working with a professional editor, they selected music to go with the tape and created a 50-minute videotape called ''Coping with Cancer.''

The group videotape experience was such a success that six or seven other adolescents in the Pediatric Oncology Clinic asked to be in the next group. Again, the new group met for six sessions, edited its own tape, put it to music, and completed a Group II version of ''Coping with Cancer.'' Since that time, five groups have gone through the process of videotaping their experiences and making educational films for the community and health professionals. Every effort is made to videotape as wide a range of the young person's activities as possible. In some of the films, we see the patients in their private moments when they ask themselves, ''Why do I have this disease?'' We travel with some of the adolescents to their schools to document their sometimes heroic efforts to be ''normal kids,'' which is the primary goal of most adolescents who carry the stigma of a serious illness. And finally, the video camera went into some of the treatment rooms and hospital wards to let others see the actual experience of treatment.

The tapes are extremely graphic in providing a sense of how adolescents feel, and how their core beliefs about themselves may have been changed by the disease. They show what some have learned from the disease, what they are able to teach others, and the techniques they use to cope with invasive procedures, such as bone marrow transplants, chemotherapy, and surgery. Very often the adolescents, in reviewing their work on the videotape, find answers to some of their own questions, and feel an enhancement of their ability to provide their own effective interventions and support when necessary. One young man who watched himself on the tape responded, ''I didn't realize I was so arrogant about my disease when I talked to other people. Maybe that's why people seem to avoid me.''

The project includes interviews with the family (parents, siblings, and grandparents) concerning their interaction with their child. They reflect on their thoughts and actions during critical periods and speak, often with telling intensity, of the stresses that affect them most. Most families and adolescents are excited about the opportunity that videotape provides to show other people "that you can have a good life even with our problem," and they enthusiastically participate in all processes of it. No videotape is made or shown without a family's permission. Although the videotapes can raise more questions than they answer, their purpose is to act as a catalyst for discussion and open nonjudgmental exploration of issues. By giving the issues a reference point in the lives of specific individuals, we hope that these groups encourage greater acceptance of the complexity of feelings that accompany the diagnosis of a life-threatening illness. This process taps into positive qualities and creativity that help create a sense of mastery and control. It is of the utmost importance that the relationship of parents and staff to the patients focuses on the strengths and positive qualities rather than on any perceived difficult behavior. It is only through this approach that adolescent patients may come more and more to value and accept themselves as individuals with control over their own lives.

One of our group members told us:

> I've really enjoyed this group. I like the fact that everybody's speaking up. It makes you feel like you're not alone. There are other people that feel the same way. It's really reassuring. You don't feel like you're left behind. There's always somebody right with you that'll stand by you, that you can relate to because you know what it feels like to get a bone marrow or what it feels like to be in a hospital to have a huge, tall, redheaded nurse. There are definitely some things I haven't talked with my parents about that I've mentioned here.
>
> This has really been a good experience. Just thinking and noticing the topics that come out. I'm not a very vocal person. I want to observe rather than talk, and I can't say it feels good to know that somebody else suffers with a bone marrow, but just the listening of this kind is support and listening to everybody's different views and giving everybody a chance to talk is so important.

It has become clear from our experience, and from the work around the country, that group work is an extremely important aspect of care of the adolescent patient (Schowalter and Lork 1970). Through group support, these patients begin to grasp the fact that their feelings are not "crazy," that there are other people who are experiencing similar things, that there are viable ways to communicate with parents, community, and caregivers, and that the word *honesty* is not just an abstract term but one that can be systematically put into practice. It is important for the staff to attempt to develop programs that are available in a particular area where a child is being treated. Treating personnel must try to remember that responses such as "My patient will never do that" or "Johnny would never participate in a group" should not deter them from making the attempt and offering the service to the child. Although being in "psychological" support work may carry a stigma in some places, we have found that someone who is offered support to help in getting through a difficult time of stress, often seizes the opportunity.

Forced Dependency

The adolescent with cancer faces an exceptional challenge in striving for independence. It is hard to feel independent when a group of strangers, known as the medical support team, give the impression that they hold your life in their hands. Adults may have preconceived expectations about how to be the "ideal patient," which usually means being passive or quiet, accepting the hospital routine with no struggle for control. The passive or depressed adolescent is usually considered the "good" patient, while the angry adolescent may be considered the "bad" patient.

> A girl diagnosed with osteogenic sarcoma had her leg amputated in an emergency procedure. The following day, she returned to the Adolescent Unit to recover from surgery. About three days later, a consultation was requested by the psychiatric oncology service because nurses and physicians noticed that she seemed excessively withdrawn and depressed. A psychologist began working with the young girl, talking to her about what it was like to lose her leg, about loss of function and her change in status in terms of her physical activity. About a week after surgery, the psychologist received an emergency call because the girl had thrown a water pitcher at one of the nurses and was calling for physicians for no apparent reason. The staff could not tolerate her angry remarks, which often had a personal, pointed quality. The psychologist met with the nurses, physicians, and parents to explain to them that her anger at this point was an extremely important channel for her resolution of grief over the loss of her leg. The parents sug-

gested that it might be best to tell her that they understood why she would be so angry, and perhaps even let her throw something against the wall to let her burn off some of the steam that had been building up. Following this communication, there was a lull in outbursts while she continued to meet with her psychologist. A couple of weeks later, when the girl had begun physical therapy, her priest came from out of state to visit her. At that point, the girl was very uncomfortable, and was learning, with the help of the parallel bars, how to balance and walk, when the priest and her parents made a surprise appearance at the Rehabilitation Department, and began to comment on how well she was doing. The girl, who was feeling extremely awkward about her recent surgery, pulled the cross off the priest's neck, threw it against the wall, and started cursing at him, telling him to leave the room. Again the psychologist received an emergency call. Again it was clear that this young girl felt justified in feeling intruded upon and also extremely angry at God. Her behavior was a way of channeling her aggression. It is important for people not to take such anger as a necessarily personal attack, although in this instance it was partly caused by a lack of respect for the patient's right to determine who might visit and when. The girl's parents were able to understand this, and also could accept that some of her anger was, in fact, not directed at them, but was a diffuse response to being in the position that she was in.

This young girl since has made an excellent recovery, is back riding a bicycle with a prosthetic device, and is a member of her junior high school swim team. Although it cannot be concluded with certainty, her ability to express her frustration, anger, and loss may have helped in her eventual good adjustment. It is our experience that adolescents who are quiet, passive, and unexpressive of underlying feelings about their disease or treatment have more difficulty in adjusting to their physical disability. It is important to understand that both anger and sadness are critical phases of the patient's and parent's experience.

Most staff working with adolescents are aware of the inevitable power struggles that are part of the adolescent's healthy quest for independence. Such questions as "Can I have the car keys tonight?" or "Why do I have to be home by 12:00?" are common in any household. For an adolescent with cancer, the treatment itself becomes the arena for such power struggles and confrontations. Fewer nonproductive struggles will occur if adolescent patients are offered, whenever possible, a wide range of options that help foster a spirit of independence by giving them some responsibility in the control of their disease. Many times, people have to tolerate deviation from strict treatment protocols. For example, adolescents can be asked which vein they prefer for an intravenous before starting chemotherapy. They can be consulted as to treatment times and schedules to avoid conflict with social events and holidays that are important aspects of their ongoing life. They can be asked to help decide as to which doctor or nurse they prefer the treatment to come from, and whether they would rather be alone or have parents or friends with them in the treatment room. One young girl, who had worked out a system of self-relaxation prior to painful procedures, became very upset when the doctor and her mother attempted to distract her during procedures. Although she felt that both of them were trying to be supportive, and she found it difficult to tell them that they were actually interfering with her method of relaxation.

The adolescent's active role in the management of the illness can be greatly enhanced by the development of skills for self-control. One potentially significant contribution to the patient's ability to increase mastery is in the area of relaxation or desensitization techniques. These techniques can be successfully employed to help deal with painful procedures. Relaxation exercises can help provide awareness of body tension and skills to reduce it. One older patient mentioned to his physician that his pain medication was not working as well as expected. He subsequently agreed to try a few relaxation exercises. He worked long hours on the procedure with his primary nurse, and finally was so satisfied with it that he began teaching his father, mother, and brother some of the skills so that they could also relax when they became tense during his treatment. The adolescent who is taught these skills develops a heightened sense of self-control. It is another area in which staff, parents, and patients can focus on some positive quality.

Reactions of Siblings

The diagnosis of cancer in the adolescent affects the whole family. For siblings, the initial period following diagnosis can be a time of confusion and fear (Kremer 1981; Sourkes 1980). Their brother or sister is acutely ill, and their parents are distracted and often absent for extended periods. Even young children sense that something is very wrong. Several measures can be helpful at this time.

Obviously, efforts should be made to try to maintain a calm atmosphere, give comfort, and provide nondisruptive care. It is equally important, despite the tendency to be totally absorbed with the sick child, that the parents place a high priority on having an honest discussion of the situation with the siblings at whatever level they may understand. Initial honesty clears the way for ongoing openness.

Siblings may be fearful that they, too, will become ill, especially if they are given blood tests. They may also feel guilty that their jealous outbursts of "Drop dead!" or "I hate you!" caused the sickness. Reassurance that they are healthy and that their feelings are normal, acceptable, and in no way cause cancer will do much to quiet these anxieties. Such constructive reassurance is possible when there is open communication among siblings, parents, and medical personnel. Creative thinking can give siblings opportunities to feel helpful. For example, when parents cannot be in the hospital, a sibling might be asked to sit with the hospitalized child to help the parents out as well as keep the patient company. Siblings also can be given assignments at home that will help the parents when they are needed in the hospital. One sibling was asked by the patient to help hang up "Get well" cards all over the wall of the hospital room so it would look like wallpaper and make the room feel like home.

Finally, when the situation has stabilized, when the weeks become months and years, siblings may come to resent the "privileged" status of the patient in the family, neighborhood, and school. Siblings are sensitive to the lack of attention to their own needs. Talking openly about society's special attentions will convince the sick person and siblings that their feelings of resentment are natural, and will enable them to share in the family crisis and encourage healthy growth and maturity. Efforts should be made to give equal attention along with explanations whenever possible. Siblings, like all children, do not care about tomorrow, but want equal treatment and attention today. It helps if one appreciates them as individuals and makes a special effort to keep in touch with their needs (American Cancer Society 1980).

Reactions of Parents

The fact that an adolescent has cancer, and the sense of being under a sentence of death, is a terrible and shocking truth for a parent to accept. Children represent our immortality; it is unthinkable that they should die before us.

Generally, it is easier at first to clutch at the straws of false hope. With hope, one wonders, "Suppose the chart has been switched or the tests misread." Somehow though, the reality of hospitalization and treatment brings the realization that the diagnosis is true. The despair that often follows such a realization can be devastating. Parents may become angry and feel defeated since their child's welfare is now dependent on someone else. They are pushed out of the parental role as primary protector and nurturer. Even worse, they feel ignorant and powerless to protect their child from the medical team and the technology that we understand only too imperfectly. In the midst of all this, there is the added burden of putting on a good front for the spouse and other family members. Moreover, the adolescent patient looks to parents for their strength in a world disrupted by unexpected and bewildering hospitalization.

All parents will go through emotionally trying times. They may have different responses. Some begin to become experts on medical information that had been incomprehensible earlier because of its unfamiliarity. Some parents become eager to learn all they can and to do whatever is asked of them, such as being part of research efforts. As the adolescent returns to health and normal vigor, the parents begin to hope that somehow their child will be the one for whom the cure works. The longer the child remains in remission, the longer the parent is allowed to cherish this hope. Despite the efforts of the team to keep the outlook realistic, parents hear about others who have lived five, ten, and even more years. They eagerly read about the new and more sensational discoveries in cancer research.

Consequently, a first relapse is apt to be even more devastating than the initial diagnosis, and many of the same feelings of guilt and despair arise. However, if the adolescent again achieves remission and returns to normal activity, the feelings of hope surface once again. Generally these feelings are tempered by the acceptance that cancer is not so easily beaten as once thought. Therefore, the family continues to seek the best treatment possible and hopes that new drugs will be found if further relapses occur (American Cancer Society 1980).

Hope seems to be a necessary component of living and not a disavowal of the fact that death is inevitable for everyone. The family of the adolescent with cancer faces the reality that anyone may die at any moment. The realization that they cannot depend on the future may inspire the family to use each moment allotted to the fullest extent. One hopes that the parent and family can learn not to wait to share themselves, their talents, and emotions until the right or convenient time. This experience with cancer can be an intensely positive experience, teaching the value of life in every moment (American Cancer Society 1980).

Why Me?

A parent might ask, "Why is my child having to go through this? Did I have some bad genes in my family? Was I too strict with my child? Did I not show enough feeling when I was raising him? Did I buy some bad food in the supermarket?" These are all questions that go through parents' minds when their adolescent is diagnosed with cancer. Frequently, the parents will also hear their child despondently ask, "Why me? Why did I have to get this disease? Why should other people have it so easy, and I have to struggle every inch of the way?" Although parents and the patient can look for spiritual, physical, and environmental reasons to try to determine the etiology of cancer, there does not appear to be any real concrete answer. What is important for the parent and the adolescent to know is that they have a right to express their feelings and anger. Parents and adolescents in our groups often address this issue:

> You have to find somebody to blame it on. It could be God; it could be the factory down the street throwing out all that junk into the air. All you can say is, I got shafted and I can't do anything about it.

Or:

> The deal of being sick; everytime you have to have treatments and you get sick, you think, "Why?" and you know if

you don't get the treatments, you're gonna die. So you feel like you're getting the needle. I don't know. I feel cheated. I feel like I'm being punished or something but not by the doctors. It's by somebody higher. The doctors are here to help us.

One teenager had this to say:

When I get up to heaven, I'm gonna ask God why we're all having to go through this, and if he doesn't give me a good answer, I'm gonna punch him right in his face, if I can.

A young girl put it this way:

Sometimes I wonder why I've had this disease, and then I begin to think about, well, this gets back to the reincarnation thing, maybe in my past life I was healthy and kind of scornful to those people that were sick, and now I'm going through this. I've really learned a lot since I've had cancer.

Most patients and parents need the space to be able to express these concerns without feeling that they are just sorry for themselves. As the young girl quoted in the foregoing expressed it in her last sentence, "I've really learned a lot since I've had cancer." The "Why me?" question is one that will never be answered fully. It is important, however, despite the devastating impact of the illness, that this question is not excessively dwelled upon. One 14-year-old girl with acute lymphocytic leukemia said, "Sometimes when I ask, 'Why me?' I say, 'Why am I so lucky?' Since I've been treated for the last ten years, I've seen kids in the clinic who have come in, been diagnosed, and have died since I've been there, and I guess sometimes I say to myself 'Why have I made it so long?' "

Summary

Illness and hospitalization can remove the adolescent from the normal social environment, family, peers, and daily activities. In addition, restrictions on mobility, physical and psychological dependency, invasion of privacy, and threats to sexuality impede attainment of crucial tasks of this age.

Adolescents respond to illness, disability, and fear in different ways. Some may withdraw, blame others, blame themselves, act more childish, or become precociously wise and mature. The likelihood of a positive adjustment is increased when the adolescent cancer patient is provided the opportunity for control and self-determination, continued reassurance about body image, and positive social interaction and restoration of self-worth.

An important consideration for professionals is to think in terms of helping the adolescent become involved in "therapeutic life-oriented programs." These programs can provide the framework for a milieu in which adolescents can ventilate and work through their anxieties, reaffirm peer group acceptance through social and recreational interaction, and constructively resume independence and control through achievements in various activity programs. These programs are offered in a variety of settings, such as patient discussion groups, music therapy, creative writing, career planning workshops, relaxation and distraction training, video production, self-help groups, and individual counseling. Sibling groups and workshops are becoming a more important area of intervention throughout the country.

We must not look at and treat patients according to how much life they have left—an evaluation that is purely a guess at best. Rather, we must help the adolescent with cancer at whatever point the patient is at physically. We must view our success as staff and parent in terms of the adolescent's own personal quality of life (Plumb and Holland 1974). Illness, change, and crisis are not easy for anyone to go through. Some months after therapy and two months before she died, a 14-year-old patient wrote this poem. Its title is "Changes."

> *People change every year.*
> *Just like you and I sitting here.*
> *These changes appear very rare.*
> *Sometimes they need special care.*
> *At times we don't like the way we change.*
> *Sometimes it seems very strange.*
> *Next time I feel a little strange,*
> *I will know it's just another change.*

References

AMERICAN CANCER SOCIETY: *Parent's Handbook, Rhode Island Hospital* (1980).

DANIEL, W. A.: *The adolescent patient.* St. Louis: Mosby, 1970.

ERIKSON, E.: *Childhood and society.* New York: Norton, 1950.

HOFFMAN, A. D., AND BECKER R. D.: Psychotherapeutic approaches to the physically ill adolescent. *Int. J. of Child Psychother.* 2 (1973): 492.

KELLERMAN, J., AND KATZ, E.: The adolescent with cancer: Theoretical, clinical and research issues. *J. of Pediatr. Psychol.* 2 (1977), no. 3: 127–131. 1977.

KOOCHER, G. P., AND O'MALLEY, J. E.: *Damocles syndrome: psychological consequences of surviving childhood cancer,* San Francisco: McGraw-Hill, 1981.

KREMER, R. F.: Living with childhood cancer: Healthy siblings' perspective, *Iss. Comp. Pediatr. Nurs.* (May 1981): 155–165.

PFEFFERBAUM, B., AND LEVENSON, P. M.: Adolescent cancer patient and physician responses to a questionnaire on patient concerns. *Am. J. Psychiatry* 139 (1982): 348–351.

PLUMB, M., AND HOLLAND, J.: Cancer in adolescents: The symptom is the thing. In B. Schoenberg, A. Carr, A. H. Kutscher, D. Peretz, I. Goldberg, (Eds.), *Anticipatory grief.* New York: Columbia University Press, 1974.

SCHOWALTER, J., AND LORK, R.: Utilization of patient meetings on an adolescent ward. *Psychiatry Med.* 1 (1970): 197–206.

SOURKES, B.: Siblings of the pediatric cancer patient. In J. Kellerman (Ed.), *Psychological aspects of childhood cancer.* Springfield, Ill.: Charles C Thomas, 1980.

TANNER, J. M.: *Growth at adolescence,* 2nd ed. Oxford: Blackwell, 1962.

VAN EYS, J.: The outlook for the child with cancer, *J. of School Health* (Mar. 1977): 165–169.

CHAPTER 3

The Adult

How PATIENTS MANAGE the diagnosis and treatment of cancer depends not only upon their inner resources but also on the support of others around them. This chapter discusses some of the issues confronting adults diagnosed with cancer and their families. It also illustrates how the professional can support the patient at the time of crisis and help the patient strive for understanding and growth even in the face of life-threatening illness. No single chapter on the adult oncology patient could provide a comprehensive review of this area. Instead, we address a selected number of common clinical problems and issues.

As medical therapies continue to lengthen the survival time of patients with cancer, the quality of survival and the emotional consequences of the illness and its treatment become more important. While many assume that distress associated with cancer is due only to physical factors, it is now apparent that much distress involves emotional and social adjustment to the disease. Some form of psychological adjustment must be faced by every patient and family dealing with the diagnosis of cancer. The development of a systematic approach to psychosocial distress in cancer patients

40

has been unduly hampered by the general view that significant depression or anxiety is a *natural* part of the disease. The question "Wouldn't you be depressed or anxious if you had cancer?" frequently functions as a disclaimer of the need for closer evaluation of the patient's situation. Until recently, there has been little formal research on the psychosocial aspects of cancer; however, an ongoing collaboration among the fields of nursing, social work, psychology, and psychiatry is beginning to generate systematic observations and increasingly reliable information.

The first step in evaluating the psychosocial situation of patients with cancer involves understanding the many medical factors that can lead directly or indirectly to difficulties in adjustment. For example, in many cases, depressive symptoms can resolve after the identification and correction of some underlying medical abnormality (see chapters 4, 5, 6). Often times, no contributing medical factor can be identified or the difficulty in adjustment continues in some form after all medical factors are dealt with as completely as possible. In these instances, we have found several issues to be so common among cancer patients that they merit general review. Some of these issues have no easy solution, but willingness to acknowledge them is often enough to decrease some of the suffering involved.

The issues addressed in this chapter include:

- Feelings of loss of control when the diagnosis of cancer is made.

- The difficulties associated with physical changes as a result of disease or its treatments.

- The relationship of social support to health and psychosocial adjustment.

- Possible interventions that lead to a more comprehensive approach to care for patients and their families.

Loss of Control

Many patients with serious illness feel a loss of control. With cancer, this feeling can be even more acute. Loss of control is inherent in the disease in that one loses control of the body's very cells. For many, the diagnosis of cancer means death. Needless to say, the disease often elicits a sense of helplessness; patients feel controlled by external forces (Miller et al. 1976). As mentioned in the previous chapter, control problems may be magnified for adolescents since issues of control for them represent a developmental task as well as a treatment issue.

For many families facing cancer, a sense of loss of control may be the critical factor precipitating distress. Difficulties in defining the disease and the extent of its treatment, as well as its duration, create the atmosphere of a sickness that has no specific beginning and no specific end. Furthermore, patients and families feel there is little they can do to stop the onslaught of a disease that often has an unclear prognosis and variable response to treatment. Unlike the situation for people with heart disease, who can at least feel effective by changing dietary, exercise, and smoking habits, there seems to be a less definitive impact of such patient-regulated activities. Curtailment of everyday functioning and ambiguity over future vocational and personal goals also contribute to feeling out of control. To be cut off suddenly from a career and the structure it provided can be a devastating blow to any patient, as this case shows:

> A 35-year-old refrigeration electrician, who was diagnosed with carcinoma of the lung, had developed spinal cord pressure that made him paraplegic. One of the most difficult things for this young man to accept, aside from the fact that he could not walk, was that he could no longer perform some of his professional responsibilities and continue the work for which he had been trained and at which he had been extremely successful. When a consultation was made to the psychiatry service, it became clear that this man could benefit from an intervention beyond simply letting him express his feelings about the loss of the use of his legs and grieving for that loss. In addition, it became evident that there were tasks he could do, related to his work, that could help make him feel more whole again. The staff encouraged various partners in his company to bring him complex mechanical pieces that needed repairs that could be done in the hospital or at home. In this case, the man was able to gain control over an extremely difficult disability by recognizing that many of his strengths and professional abilities were not lost to him and that he could continue his work in a meaningful way.

It is becoming more and more evident that continuation of aspects of life prior to illness is a key to psychosocial adjustment to disease and helps restore a sense of control in a very difficult situation.

Patients need to be given appropriate opportunities to exercise some form of control over their therapy and environment. Information about diagnosis and treatment creates such an opportunity for most people. Although withholding the diagnosis from patients may be less common than in the past (see chapter 9), it still occurs. This practice deprives the patient and the family of the opportunity to share responsibility and conveys a covert message that all control is lost. Such adverse consequences are demonstrated by the following case:

> A 32-year-old woman was diagnosed with Ewing sarcoma. Her husband, in an attempt to protect her from severe emotional strain, arranged to have the diagnosis kept from her. He convinced the physician to explain to her only that she had a rare bone disease and needed treatment with various kinds of drugs. When the physician told her that one of the side effects of the drugs would be hair loss, she started screaming and began kicking the doctor. A year later, in discussing what she had been through during that first year before she finally learned what the diagnosis was, she expressed the belief that if she had been told initially what the treatments were for and why, for example, she had to lose her hair, she would have found it much easier to handle the situation. She also wished she could have avoided the embarrassment of her earlier behavior.

Intellectual mastery can be an important means of asserting control. Gerle et al. (1960) reported that giving a group of cancer patients all the facts about their illness resulted in considerably less anxiety and depression, with a resultant decrease in the use of psychotropic drugs, compared with a group given little or no information. While blatant withholding may be rare (as in the preceding case), it is not uncommon for families to request that oncologists withhold the specific diagnosis from elderly patients. It is important for the psychosocial team (see chapter 8) to be sensitive to this kind of request. It may be symptomatic of deeper communication issues in the family system that need further intervention. To become active participants, the family and the patient need information regarding disease, treatment, home health care management, and possible future psychosocial problems. The sense of mastery engendered by knowledge increases personal control and minimizes the helplessness cycle noted by numerous researchers as being a source of depression and chronic illness.

The American Cancer Society has developed programs throughout the country to increase patients' and families' knowledge and sense of control over the disease. "I can cope" groups, which began in the Minnesota American Cancer Society, have now spread throughout the United States. They offer various workshops on medical aspects of the disease, discuss issues concerning body changes and social supports, and provide open-ended forums for patients to address questions to professionals about what to expect and what is being experienced during the course of the disease. Some families and patients can overcome their loss of a sense of control by acting as teachers or leaders for other patients in sharing information on how to overcome barriers. "Reach for recovery" and "I can cope" are both excellent examples of how experienced patients can speak to other patients to prepare them for what they will go through during the disease and in terms of their treatments. For other resources, providers may consult a recent review of major regional and national services targeted at persons with cancer, their families, and their friends (Blumberg and Flaherty 1980).

Other ways to help patients maintain a sense of competence and control are to encourage continued involvement in domestic and financial matters, to teach them self-regulatory behavioral methods such as self-relaxation to decrease side effects of drugs, or even on day-to-day issues, give them the opportunity to select the veins in which to start intravenous lines.

Self-care is another way to encourage patients to avoid the regression associated with illnesses. This method is being tried in various inpatient settings. It has always been a common practice for nurses to make the bed and to bathe, and often feed, adult patients who are hospitalized for fairly long periods of time while receiving treatment. There is increasing recognition of the value of involving patients in self-care, for example, by making their own beds or straightening up their rooms. Eating in group meal situations increases socializing on the floor and, by taking more control over their own care, patients reduce the feeling of helplessness. Assuming reasonable responsibility for active participation in one's own health care is extremely valuable. With it comes an increased sense of control over one's fate and a lessening of the feeling of helplessness that often accompanies the disease. Attempts to assert some control are often found at the core of patients' and families' angry reactions, noncompliance, and antitherapeutic behavior. A change of attitude often follows a change of role from that of passive victim to active participant.

Physical Changes

Loss of body integrity or a body part causes a grief situation often characterized by typical signs and symptoms of severe psychological distress. Well-intentioned remarks to an individual—such as, "Lighten up, you'll get over it"—communicate that the painful psychological issues associated with a sense of damage and physical body image change are unimportant or should be ignored. However, the sharing of emotional reactions to loss is an important part of grief resolution. The problems of coping with physical loss are mostly determined by the private meaning the loss has for the individual patient. Providers should not assume that each individual reacts to loss in a predictable way, but should ask questions that allow patients to reveal their own private issues.

Physical loss also will affect different individuals for different reasons. A pro football player who is injured diving into a shallow swimming pool will react very differently than a lawyer whose mind is left intact and who has never depended on physical prowess for success. Some questions that open up this area are "What was it like for you to hear about needing surgery?" or "What sort of difficulties are you having at home now?" or "What has been the most difficult part of your treatment to adjust to?"

Physical loss can lead to new problems with mobility, self-care, and role function that in themselves can create feelings of helplessness and isolation if not concretely addressed by using available rehabilitative resources. It is important that the caregiver realize that each disease and treatment modality may be associated with unique concerns and rehabilitative issues.

Mental health providers should make themselves aware of the disease-specific rehabilitation issues faced by patients. For example, patients receiving radiotherapy may worry about being burned or losing sexual function (Rotman et al. 1977). Breast cancer patients also have their unique concerns (Silberfarb 1978; Schain 1976), including such phenomena as "phantom" sensations of the missing breast (Jarvis 1967) that seldom would be discussed unless specifically asked about. While there have been few formal studies of the subject, the prevalence of sexual dysfunction associated with cancer appears to be significant and should be an important area of concern for the caregiver. Although the incidence of sexual dysfunction approaches 100% in women who have cancer affecting genital organs (Jewett 1975; VonEschenbach 1980; Dempsey et al. 1975; Donahue et al. 1977), the problem is *not* limited to genital cancers. Derogatis and Kourlesis (1981) have written an excellent review article on this area, which should be required reading for providers.

It is important for the family to recognize that the loss of a body function from an amputation or of hair from chemotherapy, or difficulty in maintaining physical stamina, are severe losses in and of themselves. This loss is often accompanied by a grief process that is very similar to the experience of losing a loved one through death. Issues such as denial, anger, bargaining, depression, and acceptance are emotional responses experienced by the grieving individual. We feel it is important for the staff to encourage the family and the patient to allow the grief to be expressed. Individual psychological responsiveness varies, of course. The family that feels and expresses the pain is often able to move beyond it and adjust to a disease or major physical loss.

Although the field of rehabilitation psychology was developed more than 60 years ago, the issues and interventions of rehabilitation are still new to the field of cancer therapy (Cromes 1978; McAleer and Kluge 1978). Disability that the cancer patient might face can be classified as either acute or chronic. Acute disabilities are often found immediately in the postoperative period where there is increased immobilization, and include fear, pain, and possible confusion on the part of both the patient and the family. Chronic disability is found where there is a potentially long-term handicap, such as with the loss of a limb due to cancer surgery. Realistic goals and program planning for the patient and the family can and should begin prior to the development of the chronic disability. Lack of adequate preparation typically is associated with poor outcome, as seen in the following case.

A 45-year-old woman patient was diagnosed with osteogenic sarcoma of the arm. No rehabilitation plans were developed before extensive surgery was completed. After the surgery, when the patient returned to the hospital bed and realized that she had lost an arm, she was extremely depressed and panicky about her future inability to care for her household and family and to maintain a sense of control over her life. She shared her extreme stress, in crying episodes, with the nurses. She expressed her fear of an extreme loss of control because of her present state and could not see any promising or corrective future.

In this case, it would have been easy to avoid postoperative panic by offering a rehabilitation intervention before the surgery. The patient could have been informed about the many alternatives and possibilities for maintaining a normal life-style at home. It has also been extremely valuable for such patients to speak with others who have undergone the amputation procedure, and have in many ways completed their rehabilitation process. It must be remembered that the psychological problems of the patient and family as a result of a physical amputation sometimes can be worse than the physical consequences of the disease itself. Therefore, the attention of the treatment team should be focused on the psychological, as well as physical and vocational, rehabilitation needs of the family unit and the patient.

It is an understatement to say that job placement and the continuation of a vocation or career for the patient with a disability can be extremely difficult. As with our earlier case of the refrigeration electrician, a positive understanding is needed by the employer to correct problems of acceptance of the employee's potential difficulties. Planning for the use of public transportation, presenting oneself for job interviews, and job placement within the limitations of the disability are important needs to be addressed by the patient and the family to alter the effects and potential complex reactions that many of these patients will experience (Dietz 1973). The complexities of the rehabilitation task can be met only by a multidisciplinary approach (Harvey et al. 1982).

Issues of Social Support

Consistent with Mechanic's summary statement (1974) that "the ability of persons to maintain psychological comfort will depend not only on the intrapsychic resources, but also—and perhaps more importantly—on the social supports available or absent in the environment," we feel that effective social support is a crucial factor in the psychosocial adaptation to cancer.

For most people, love and supportive relationships provide the underlying strength and framework for meeting the challenges of life and death. A stable relationship that meets emotional needs provides a refuge and secret source of strength in times of trouble. Yet even a cursory view of our current cultural trends reveals that the organization of traditional support structures has been disrupted. Geographic mobility, rising divorce rates, decentralization of the family, and new life-style patterns all contribute to fragmentation of social support systems. The phenomenal rise of social programs attests to the fact that institutions and agencies have become necessary to fulfill supportive roles once the responsibility of family and community.

There has been increasing research documenting the fact that a relative lack of social support is a factor in both the onset and adaptation to medical disorders. The recognition and investigation of the impact of the social system on health have been a basic sociologic issue since Durkeim's (1951) pioneering study on social integration and suicide over 70 years ago. As Cassel (1974) has pointed out, the epidemiologic perspective of the genesis of disease has increasingly come to take social factors into account along with the biologic and psychological. There has been extensive general documentation linking periods of illness to stresses, including disturbed social relations (Dohrenwend and Dohrenwend 1981). In terms of a derived explanatory model, it has been suggested that disturbed social relations create a stress that may lead to a weakened physical state and increased illness vulnerability. Social support is also thought to mediate psychological distress, facilitate coping and adaptation (Andrews et al. 1978), and thereby alter physiologic vulnerability and illness. The dozens of studies directed toward investigating this model have been exhaustively reviewed (Kaplan et al. 1977). In an excellent review of the effects of social support, Heller (1978) has pointed out:

> While the importance of group ties no longer is in dispute, it is time to go beyond the simple truism that social support has been beneficial, to an examination of the conditions and mechanisms by which social support operates most optimally. In order to clarify the active factors in the support phenomenon, skilled research is needed in which support programs are tested in controlled demonstration projects. Such research can provide a bridge between hypothesis and application. Such a bridge is

crucial in the development of improved care programs for the terminally ill.

While it is currently held that social support may provide a mediating influence between individuals and their ability to cope with or adapt to stressful situations, there has been no universal agreement on a definition of social support or its measurement. In general, the development of the concept and measurement of social support begins at a simple demographic level and moves toward more subjective perceptions of social support network. More important than the number of people available is some factor of the qualitative nature of the relationships (Berkman 1977; Brown et al. 1975). The two basic properties of social support systems are their *morphology* and their *interactional properties*. Morphology consists of four factors: the number of supports, the accessibility of supports, the connectedness of supports, and the immediacy of contacts. The interactional properties of support include the meanings that persons in the network give to the relationships, the amount of reciprocity in the relationship, the intensity of the relationship, and the frequency of the relationship. This basically derives from Mitchell's Social Network Theory (1969), a review and summary of the concept of social support. Cobb (1976) has organized the various aspects of support into four categories: social, instrumental, active, and material support. *Material support* relates to goods and services. *Active support* refers to mothering—what mothers do for infants, or what nurses do for patients. *Instrumental support* refers to counseling. *Social support* is purely informational and has three components—emotional support (leading the recipient to believe that he or she is cared for and loved), esteem support (leading the recipient to believe that he or she is esteemed and valued), and network support (leading the recipient to believe that he or she is in a defined position in a network of communication and mutual obligation).

Both Mitchell and Cobb highlight one important factor that is generally absent in measures of social support—the factor of "reciprocity." Simply stated, each person has different needs for social support. Some individuals might function quite well with very little support, while for others the needs may be overwhelming. It would seem that the relationship betweeen needs and supplies is probably a more useful measure than either alone. This relationship has been called a "person–role fit" (French et al. 1974). An instrument designed to assess the informational aspect of social support in terms of a person–environment fit has been developed by Ann Kaplan (1977). Recognition of this reciprocal nature of social support represents an important methodological advance.

In addition to playing an important role in maintaining psychological well-being (Turner 1981), social support may influence both the quality of survival and its length. Using information from psychological autopsies of cancer deaths, and correlations of observed survival (measured in months beyond expected survival) with psychosocial findings, Weisman and Worden (1975) found that patients who lived significantly longer tended to maintain cooperative and mutually responsive relationships, especially toward the end of their lives. Patients with death wishes, depression, apathy, and long-standing mutually destructive relationships survived for shorter periods than expected. Why longevity occurs in some patients, but not in others, may be related to different traits that create alienation in personal life and in caretaking staff as life draws to a close. More assertive patients may ask for and get better attention and services, and a result, may live longer and die better deaths.

Cancer often brings with it a loss of social acceptability, isolation, and a sense of abandonment, all of which can become significant sources of difficulty for the patient. For a variety of reasons, friends, relatives, and employers may withdraw from the patient. (Abrams 1966). Many people assume that cancer is contagious and therefore avoid contact with a patient for fear of contamination. Employers may be reluctant to rehire cancer patients because they fear prolonged absences due to treatments or they assume the employee will be alive only for a short period of time. Most people are uncomfortable with the prospect of facing a cancer patient because of fears of their *own* mortality. Even well-meaning family members may not be able to provide effective support because of the problems of not knowing what to talk about during a visit. Such questions arise as: Should I talk about the illness? Should I ask how the patient is feeling? Should I ask how the patient is coping? What can I do to help this person and offer support at this most difficult time? There are various ways of helping significant others provide effective support. For example, public education could potentially provide information to demystify the disease and the treatments for it. Several comprehensive source books of information and education material have been made available by the National Cancer Institute (NIH Publication no. 80–2129, 80–2080, 81–2059), along with many other materials on various diseases and treatments. During a difficult treatment regimen, patient and family often back off from their regular contacts, work, and relationships. Although the mechanical aspects of this withdrawal often are unavoidable because of the treatments, it is important for staff to help the patient and family assess their priorities for staying involved in various community activities and employment. Concrete assistance, such as through a homemaker, babysitter, visiting nurse, or financial assistant, may help the family manage at home and maintain important social networks when things otherwise seem overwhelming.

The challenge to the cancer patient often becomes finding a reason "why" to live in order to find a way "how" to live. The "whys" in life vary. For some people, the "why" is relationships, caring, and friendship. For others, it is money or career. And for others, it may be some cause or religion or people. We all need a reason to exist. However, when confronted with a life-threatening illness, our reason for existence may shift. Such illness makes one question all of those reasons, as seen in the following case:

> A middle-aged husband and father of a young child was diagnosed with Hodgkin's disease. Because of his academic needs as a psychologist, the couple had always moved to cities where there was employment despite their lack of the kind of social support system they desired. At the time of diagnosis, the family was thrown into a turmoil concerning the issue of traditional versus nontraditional treatment. Upon completion of successful radiation and chemotherapy combination, the couple (who sought help from the psychiatric service) decided that they wished to live in an area to which numerous friends and family had moved over the past years. This crisis entailed making a move without a job and created another intense situation where there would be a lack of security. Dealing with a crisis as a family helped them resolve the dilemma by moving to where they would be able to share one full-time job. They made a major life-style change in terms of spending more time with their child and with each other, and of being in a place where they had long wished to be.

It is important for the family facing the diagnosis of cancer to understand that having a life-threatening illness is a crisis and a time of stress in terms of social support and personal interactions and priorities. It can be an uncomfortable yet a promising time of potential growth and individual development rather than a time of failure. The major difference between this crisis and other traditional crises such as rape and divorce is that in a life-threatening crisis there is an additional component: The life/death philosophical confrontation that forces the family to confront basic life values.

The Spouse or Significant Key Other

The main burden of providing support to the adult cancer patient usually falls on the spouse or children. What is sometimes overlooked is that such persons are themselves under tremendous strain as a result of the emotional demands and new responsibilities, including managing the family, coordinating finances, and providing primary care for the patient (Wellisch et al. 1978). The loss of physical intimacy that often accompanies severe illness may leave a couple stranded from each other, if they are not accustomed to sharing their intimate feelings in other ways. As the community has difficulty with the diagnosis of cancer, well-meaning family members, even when available, either may not know how or find it very difficult to provide support to the ill family member or to feel supportive themselves in the process. A primary goal of the treatment team might be not only to provide optimum care for the individual facing the illness, but also to recognize when those who care for the patient need support. For example, the family that wishes to withhold the diagnosis from the patient is often one that can use support and help in developing communication skills and providing support for the patient in the long run. While it has been generally stated that the medical establishment is just beginning to pay proper attention to the psychosocial needs of cancer patients, even less has been done systematically to address the needs of the family. Involving the significant key other (SKO) may also be the most sensible way to help the patient cope. No professional can ever be as close to or know the patient as well as the spouse. It is also evident that the SKO is the person on whom the patient relies most in time of intense crisis. It seems to make little sense, therefore, iatrogenically to displace the spouse in favor of some professional when the patient is having a problem. In fact, it may be both more cost effective and more logical to have the SKO fill a role that is often assigned to some outside person.

The role of the SKO should be thought of as consisting of the following tasks:

1. *To help maintain the social support system of the patient.* This is always stressed and often fragmented in dying patients. Even when family and friends are nearby, the impact of cancer diagnosis often brings considerable anxiety and distress. At times, family members may avoid visiting the patient in the hospital. The SKO is often in the pivotal position of receiving information about the spouse's condition and sharing it with those concerned. It will be important for the SKO to interact with family members and friends in a manner than can help reduce anxiety and increase contact between the patient and his/her loved ones.

2. *To promote the patient's sense of autonomy.* Loss of a sense of control is a common feature for the dying and may contribute to maladaptive behaviors developed in that phase. Helping the patient maintain a sense of integrity and worth during the experience of serious disability is an important task for the SKO. It involves both interpersonal and task-related dimensions. On an interpersonal level, the verbal and/or nonverbal communication that the patient is as loved and valued as ever provides major support. In addition, being sensitive to what the patient can continue to do for him/herself will give the patient continued opportunity to experience mastery in whatever daily activities he/she can accomplish and enjoy.

3. *To be an advocate for the patient when necessary.* The goals of the biomedical treatment team may not always be congruous with patient needs. Having an awareness of the patient's ability to interact effectively with health care staff, the SKO may find that at times his/her input is necessary in providing important information to guide the treatment effectively. These activities may include communicating to treating staff about symptoms or side effects of treatment when the patient is home and not feeling up to phoning the doctor. It may also include meeting with staff and participating in decisions about when to terminate treatment. This decision can be a very personal one in which the family's values are more a determining factor than are specific medical principles. The SKO can articulate his/her values as shared by the patient and thereby help guide the treatment.

The following situation demonstrates the clinical application of using the SKO as patient advocate.

Mr. A is a 62-year-old prostatic cancer patient with bone metastases. He is in a home care program. Both the patient and the visiting nurse are frustrated by the lack of adequate analgesia. Each home visit is marked by a sense of frustration about not being able to relieve the patient's suffering and there is a growing sense of frustration with the physician, who seems distant and overly cautious. The instinct of the nurse is to point out to the physician what is happening, and insist on a change in medication. Not only can this experience be frustrating and create some tension, especially when the physician reacts defensively, but the apparent caring motivation of the nurse paradoxically can have a negative effect on the patient and family inasmuch as it displaces them from acting on their own behalf. If possible, the patient should be educated about being a more effective consumer. If the patient is having the pain, why not have the patient discuss this with the physician? The nurse could spend some time helping the patient consolidate the skills needed to do this. Or, if the patient is too weak or is ineffective for other reasons, the SKO or family can become involved as advocates for the patient. The family is looking for ways to be helpful. Here is a concrete situation in which they can do something. They will feel better, the patient will feel better, and the nurse can feel effective without confrontation.

4. *To encourage communication between the patient and family and friends.* It is generally agreed that open and honest communication is a healthier and more adaptive approach than silence when dealing with cancer (Kaplan 1981). A prevalent attitude toward patient–family communication has been stated as follows: ''If communication within the family has been open and full in the past, it will probably be maintained during the course of a terminal illness . . . the physician must assure that faulty communication does not add to the patient's burden'' (Hackett 1976). However, empirical support for such clinically sensible observations has been generally lacking. Maddison and Raphael (1972) maintain that lack of openness and restrained communications are a problem but again there are few published data demonstrating that a change in communication patterns betters the quality of life for patients or family members. One study has concluded that among the characteristics that help a family make a good adjustment to serious illness is direct and consistent communication (Olsen 1970). Krant and

Johnston (1977–1978) have looked at family members' perceptions of communication in late-stage cancer. They found that many first-order relatives did not have communication links to the physician, especially if direct communication was not established at the time of diagnosis. Intrafamilial communications regarding illness and dying were frequently discordant and guarded, leading to perceptions that the patient was withdrawing, and fostering a reliance upon the hospital for terminal care. More than half the family members reported that they were uncomfortable when visiting the patient in the hospital, experienced feelings of helplessness, or sensed significant helplessness in the patient. Bearing the patient's pain was seen as particularly difficult. Information concerning dying patients is often withheld or distorted.

In spite of a positive relationship with the patient, negative associations about the disease can create the following problems in communication: (a) Fears can arise concerning the emotional impact of disclosure of the diagnosis and prognosis to the patient. A problem of information that is common among family members but not shared is that although everyone knows, no one talks about this shared knowledge. The isolation resulting from this communication dysfunction increases stress among family members. (b) Fears about the patient's decline—anticipating pain and physical disintegration—can result in withdrawal from the patient based on the SKO's anxiety about the impending disability. (c) Fear of the contagiousness of cancer is still a prominent concern among many people. (d) There can be uncertainty about how to talk with the patient—a compulsion to try to "cheer up" the patient, while genuine sadness is being denied. This shallow approach is often experienced as nonsupportive and a break in an empathic bond. An intervention for the SKO can provide a place to review interaction difficulties and generate alternative ways to deal with communication problems. Often the chance to express fears and grief and to "practice" open discussion with a therapist frees the SKO to bring this behavior back to interaction with the patient, family members, and friends in the social network.

5. *To facilitate the expression of feeling.* This is often difficult for people around the life-threatening illness, as illustrated by the following example:

A 38-year-old married woman was diagnosed with a rare type of bone cancer after experiencing constant pain in her leg for three months. During the initial diagnosis and surgery, friends and community were very supportive of the couple, providing them with strong psychological backup and helping with tasks such as babysitting, keeping the house clean, and furnishing transportation for other children. Although the prognosis for the particular cancer was good on the basis of five-year survival rates, the couple still wondered how the wife would do over the long run and what would happen if she relapsed. When entering treatment, the couple reported extreme difficulty in deciding who was having a more difficult time with the illness. The wife felt that her husband really could not understand what it was like for her to experience the pain and fear of loss as well as the difficulty of accepting and complying with treatments. The husband felt that his wife did not know what he was experiencing in terms of anxieties about dealing with the children, fears of losing her, and the overall existential pain of living on a day-to-day basis with so much uncertainty. Both thought they were hurting more as a result of the disease. Although the wife was relatively accessible to psychological help, the husband had extreme difficulty in finding a support system where other spouses of cancer patients could talk about their feelings, be cared for by each other, and express their needs in relating to the process of the disease.

The physician sometimes can be helpful in such situations by tactfully bringing out into the open issues that seem to be hidden between a couple. At other times, the significant supporting person with major coping problems may require referral to a mental health professional. The mental health consultant who engages the SKO in counseling can gently elicit affect while respecting the individual's style of coping. Since the patient is the most dramatic focus of concern during the crisis of cancer diagnosis and treatment, the needs of the spouse or special friend are overlooked. Nevertheless, the stress involved with being the primary support of "the patient" can be overwhelming. "What can I do? I feel so helpless. I feel like I am going crazy. What is going to happen to me?" These are typical concerns. It is important to try to understand what is going on when an SKO appears to be having difficulty fulfilling his or her role.

There are six important issues that staff should be aware of when trying to understand the reasons that some SKOs have a problem in providing support:

1. The SKO must maintain a balance between being vitally involved and being able to let go. When confronted with a

terminal illness in the spouse, anticipatory grieving may begin immediately. The SKO must keep a delicate balance between pulling back prematurely and remaining so involved that the later shock of the loss is overwhelming.

2. The staff must be aware that the SKO may have physical and psychological limitations that interfere with the fulfillment of the role of "good spouse."

3. The SKO may have to alter personal life-style. For example, some may quit a job to care for the sick patient, and then face major problems in reestablishing themselves. They also may lose their own social support systems and become isolated from their usual sources of solace.

4. The SKO must face the challenge of planning for a future without the spouse, of becoming involved in unaccustomed major life tasks such as financial planning, care of the children, and redefinition as an individual rather than a couple.

5. Some SKOs might find themselves overwhelmed by the revival of past unresolved grief. This re-kindled grief can significantly interfere with how they relate to the patient.

6. The SKO may develop his/her own depressive reaction, confusion, and stress-response syndrome.

While everyone is catering to the patient's emotional and physical state, the SKO often either is ignored or is given bland reassurances and condolences that overlook internal emotional realities, as the following example illustrates:

The husband of a 52-year-old mother of three children was diagnosed with a tumor involving his spinal cord. Recovery from his initial surgery required a five-week hospital stay, which was punctuated by several medical complications. These included severe anemia that required transfusion and high fever from a surgical wound infection that required a course of intravenous antibiotics. Probably, in part, because of her professional appearance and organized style, the wife was assumed to be coping well and was generally ignored by the treatment team. While more progressive treatment teams routinely include and inform the spouse of ongoing medical issues, it may be unrealistic to assume that the spouse of every patient can be, or even needs to be, provided with a relationship to deal with his/her own emotional responses to the patient's illness. In this particular case, because of the overall competent outward appearance of the wife, she was given very little information. Her internal emotional turmoil, however, came to light through disturbing behaviors rather than by carefully chosen rational communication. The nursing staff recognized that every time she visited her husband he became more physically agitated. The initial response of the staff was to limit her visits in an effort to keep the patient calm. It should be obvious that any attempt at such a solution does not make sense before a more individualized assessment of what was going on within the person. One night, she told one of the evening nurses that she felt she was losing control, had some suicidal feelings, and required some professional help. A number of important issues finally came to light when a psychiatric consultation was finally called at her request. As it turned out, some of her own past experiences were leading to significant distortions in her perception of her husband's current situation. Specifically, she reported having one relative who had severe anemia that was finally diagnosed as due to cancer. She thus assumed that her husband's anemia was the result of another cancer that was being kept secret from her. She also reported that a relative had died following a severe infection that was treated with intravenous antibiotics. In her mind, her husband's infection was of a similar life-threatening nature and in a sense was an omen of his impending death. It was helpful to her to learn that she was confusing her experiences and that it was important to separate what had happened in the past from the reality of what was happening with her husband. With this clarification, she was able to feel much less frantic and disorganized, and her husband began to perceive her visits as more comforting and less ominous.

Fortunately, this woman was able to tell the staff what some of her needs were. In many cases, however, staff must assume the responsibility for bringing the spouse's difficulty to the attention of the treatment team. Although it is up to the family to try to let someone know what is disturbing them, physicians and nurses must be aware of the situation, and reassure the spouse and other family members that they are interested in how they are coping and that they can refer them to others who will answer questions about the patient's treatment. It must be remembered that people may not be consciously aware of such problems, and if they are, do not know how or with whom to discuss them. Also, they might feel uncomfortable in sharing their concerns with outsiders, and so not express them at all.

Spouses and family members obviously bring their own unique background experiences to the illness situation. The SKO must always be viewed as a person with an individual history, which will in part determine the capacity to be involved in the treatment process. Many of the SKOs of patients with life-threatening illness encounter significant difficulty with relationships, communication, and affective responses with which they might be helped in some manner by a counselor or therapist. However, unless the counselor or therapist is aware of the unique issues inherent in the SKO's position, the intervention may not take place at all. The foremost goal of the counselor is creation and maintenance of a relationship in which the SKO can better deal with the stresses, challenges, and supportive tasks involved with caring for a patient with cancer.

The relevant techniques for counseling SKOs have been systematized as part of a project of one of the authors (Goldberg and Wool 1982). In this project it was found the SKOs were quite variable, depending on personality style, defenses, and expectations. The "ideal" SKO for counseling is one who is psychologically oriented, has some general understanding of the parameters of the counselor–client relationship, recognizes the special stresses created by the current life crisis, and feels positive about obtaining some relief by talking about the experience, even though such an undertaking might itself be emotionally difficult. In reality, most SKOs differ from the ideal composite in one or all of these parameters. Because SKOs are often not self-selected or self-referred "counseling" candidates, they may not be psychologically oriented and be unaccustomed to a one-to-one relationship in which personal, private issues are discussed. They may be actively denying the impact of the life-threatening illness, or frightened about getting in touch with their responses to it. And they may undervalue or have distorted fantasies about what it means to be in a counseling relationship. The perception of such issues by the counselor and the ways of managing them constitute a specific counseling approach. The following case is an example of the resolution of a communication problem and illustrates the usefulness of historical inquiry, such as what the role the SKO played in getting the patient involved in treatment, since events from that phase of illness may be important in later adjustment.

He was coughing for so many years I just gave up talking about it but now I feel guilty about the decision to delay seeing a doctor. I was so afraid underneath about what they might find that I kept finding reasons for him not to see the doctor. Now I wonder what he is thinking about me and I am too uncomfortable to go see the doctor with him now.

The SKO's perception of this role in the onset of illness may be an important factor to address explicitly. For some, it is may be helpful to assist in rationalizing events. Clearly, physical symptoms such as coughing are so common that it would be impossible to bring each instance to medical attention. Preoccupation with illness can be a disabling disease in itself, and paradoxically often leads to misdiagnosis since physicians may stop listening to those who lose their credibility. Most often, we say "that cough always goes away after a while," or conclude that for "the pain in my leg must be from the weather, or perhaps I bumped it somewhere." The need to deny the potential danger of the warning signals of cancer can lead intelligent people to appear unabashedly naive: "I can get that sore on my back to stop bleeding if I don't wear a shirt like this anymore." Our need to see ourselves and our loved ones as healthy may lead us to downplay the potential reasons for symptoms. Such benign neglect usually proves to be appropriate, but sometimes it leads to delay in diagnosis. Such a delay can make a person who knew of the symptoms but did not press the patient to seek medical advice feel guilty and unrealistically responsible for someone else's disease. It may be important to help the SKO share such a concern with the patient. Often this leads to the discovery that the patient is genuinely not intent on blaming the SKO. But if this is an issue, it is better brought out into the open since unspoken and distorted blame and guilt can poison a relationship that cannot afford such a secret burden. Sometimes, no matter what is said, the patient and significant other will continue to feel blame and guilt, which may reflect a long-standing marital dynamic. Therefore, any assessment of difficulties between the patient and SKO must be measured against their baseline adjustment.

Unfortunately life is too complex to permit the formulation of a simple recipe that one might follow to be a more effective significant key other. Individual needs of patients and SKOs, as well as unique characteristics of the relationship and the situation, make for a huge number of possible variables. No one rule is right for everyone. However, the issues raised here may help the professional gain some perspective concerning the problem facing the spouse and the patient.

Psychosocial Interventions

As stated throughout the book, the intervention with adult cancer patients is a relatively new field that has just recently become more developed. It is not uncommon to attend a lecture on the psycho-social aspects of cancer and to hear described extremely elaborate intervention programs devised for those facing malignancy in childhood. It is also extremely common for members of the audience to raise the question, "What about adults?" The mechanics of providing psychological interventions for adult cancer patients are more difficult than for children because their number is so much higher. Yet there are many options and programs that can be developed in small or large hospitals to provide more supportive care for the family facing cancer. Thus far, much of the research involving long-term survivors of cancer also has been done in the pediatric area. Only now are researchers and clinicians beginning to consider the psychological aspects of long-term survivors in adult cancer.

The psychosocial impact of cancer on the patient has been described in a number of papers (Peck 1972; Craig and Abeloff 1974; Freidenbergs et al. 1979; Maguire et al. 1978; Morris et al. 1977; Plumb and Holland 1981), with some overall agreement that anxiety and depression are clinically relevant symptoms in about one third of patients. Furthermore, there is some evidence to indicate that such symptoms are not limited to the "crisis" phase around the time of diagnosis but may remain active for months (Gottesman and Lewis 1982), or up to one year (Maguire et al. 1978; Morris et al. 1977) after initial diagnosis. Despite the long-standing and generally accepted recognition of the presence of significant psychosocial distress associated with cancer, it is only recently that there have been any systematic and methodologically acceptable efforts to develop, deliver, and evaluate a psychosocial intervention designed specifically for cancer patients. While there seems to be a great deal of literature devoted to counseling for death and dying (Weisman 1972; Kübler-Ross 1969; Fiefel 1977; Kastenbaum and Aisenburg 1976; Schneidman 1976), there are relatively few contributions delineating tested interventions for problems associated with surviving with cancer. Even before applying any intervention, however, it is necessary first, of course, to identify the patients with actual or potential problems. Screening for high-risk and high-symptom-level patients is especially important as there could never be enough resources (nor would it be clinically appropriate) to intervene with every cancer patient. Project Omega, an extended longitudinal research project at Massachusetts General Hospital under the aegis of Doctors A. D. Weisman and J. W. Worden, has provided some important contributions in the area of screening patients for risk for psychosocial morbidity (Weisman and Worden 1980). As of yet, there are no generally agreed upon and easily administered methods to identify the population at risk for significant psychosocial problems.

These investigators also have addressed the important question, "Do cancer patients really want counseling?" (Worden and Weisman 1980). One third of the newly diagnosed cancer patients, which they screened to be at high risk, refused a counseling intervention. Refusers tended to be more antagonistic and apprehensive than those who accepted. Refusers tended to deny difficulties and to minimize problems, and in certain instances were truculent and suspicious. Some refused for fear that their social and emotional equilibrium might be disturbed; they rejected counseling as an immediate threat or an implication of disaster. It is important that these factors be realized by anyone who wishes to apply counseling intervention to cancer patients. Such patients are not "psychiatric" patients. They do not view their problem as necessarily having a psychologic component, and are often not self-referred. These factors raise special issues that the counselor must be prepared to address if engagement of an "at-risk" patient is to be successful. While there may be some "hard" refusers who are impossible to engage under any circumstances, there is no doubt a middle ground group or "soft" refusers where clinical skill will make the difference as to whether they engage or remain involved in an intervention or not. Despite fears of some providers to the contrary, the *majority* of patients agree to accept a psychosocial intervention, and even among the refusers, some can probably be engaged over time. Knowing that most cancer patients would agree to a psychosocial intervention, the next question to consider is, "Has there been any demonstration that it can make a difference?" For example, it would have been interesting to follow the psychosocial course of Worden and Weisman's acceptance and refusal groups to see if the offered counseling mattered. Several studies have undertaken the difficult and complex challenge to demonstrate the effects of psychosocial intervention. Gorden et al. (1980) have evaluated the effect of a psychosocial intervention program on psychosocial problems in patients with breast cancer, lung cancer, and melanoma. Using a control group, they demonstrated that their intervention effectually ameliorated some of the psychosocial problems reported by patients, and the intervention patients were more likely to return to work, to be more active, and to have fewer mood disturbances.

Forester et al. (1982) reported a decrease in dysphoric mood as well as physical symptoms associated with radiotherapy for patients given 30 minutes of weekly psychotherapy over six weeks of treatment. Capone et al. (1980) investigated the effectiveness of in-hospital individual counseling on the psychosocial adjustment of patients with newly diagnosed gynecologic malignancies. Levels of psychologic distress, sexual functioning, and return to employment were assessed at three, six, and 12 months after counseling. Compared with the control group, the counseled group had better function on all outcome measures. Linn et al. (1982) tested the effect of a counseling intervention on quality of survival, functional status, and length of survival of 120 terminal cancer patients in the first randomized prospective study of its kind. The experimental group was found to improve significantly more than the controls on quality-of-life measures. Other pilot studies are taking place that explore whether a psychological intervention can influence the actual physical progression of the illness (Simonton et al. 1980).

Because of funding difficulties in the area of chronic illness and psychological adaptation, it is extremely difficult to initiate programs for the support of cancer patients in various hospital settings. Therefore, there is a great need to create innovative cost-effective programs that can be implemented in a variety of cancer care settings. To develop such programs, there is a need further to define the at-risk groups and to concentrate on brief, group, or systems interventions.

At Rhode Island Hospital, the Psychiatry Department implemented a program that assigned a psychologist to assess the needs and the resources available in the hospital and in the community in providing support for cancer patients and their families. Through this, the department was able to coordinate a number of existing personnel, including mental health, physical therapy, nursing, and other involved professionals who were dealing with cancer patients, to meet on a regular basis to discuss some of the issues they faced in providing care for their patients. The goal of this meeting was to assess the needs of various services as well as to decrease the psychosocial problems related to the chronic illness. Components frequently addressed included physician–patient relationships, nurse–patient relationships, issues of open communication with the family, increased participation of the family in care, assessment of skill building and crisis management, and provision of mutual support to others and maintenance of normality in terms of vocational and home functioning. One of the problems that became clearer as a result of this meeting was the fact that many oncologists and nurses tended to be extremely protective and discouraged outside help for their patients.

As psychosocial interventions are developed for individuals and families with cancer, the key to their success will depend not only on the specific training of the professional, but, more important, also on the attitude of the oncologist and the cancer nurse toward identifying and addressing patient needs. As long as clinicians maintain the assumption that depression, anxiety, and difficulty in adjusting to cancer are normal and do not necessarily need professional support, psychosocial needs will remain unmet.

Individualized Family Teaching Plan

One of the more basic interventions that an oncology service should strive for is a comprehensive, individualized teaching plan that can be developed to ensure that families receive the information they need for informed decision making and participation in their own health care. The teaching plan can be placed in as simple a format as a check-list and may consist of specific behavioral objectives to be achieved. Among the areas that this plan might encompass could be diagnosis, family conference follow-up sessions for answering questions, review of various written materials from either the local hospital or the American Cancer Society related to the individual disease, and individual teaching sessions on the disease, treatment procedures, blood counts, and psychosocial issues in home care management. To address the specific problems that develop for each individual patient or family, there might be specifically and appropriately timed programs covering topics such as late effects of treatment, terminal care and bereavement, bone transplants, and bone marrow transplantation. As a result of the recent boom in video equipment and productions, it is not difficult for most hospital settings to develop the visual materials that are available to patients, families, friends, and staff. Various tapes can be used to reinforce teaching, provide for special population needs, and allow for flexible learning experiences. For example, one tape was developed that discussed the psychological issues that face women when they go through a mastectomy. On the tape are group discussions by women who have been through the procedure, indicating how they coped with it and what some of the special problems are, and describing some of the various drugs and treatments used throughout the course of the illness. The value of these videotapes is that they are accessible to patients to watch whenever they feel the need to have questions answered and there is no staff around. Such tapes should supplement, not replace, staff contact, of course.

Groups

The formation of support groups for adults and families with cancer is neither surprising nor new because of the tendency for people with common problems to unite for their common good. The impetus for program development often comes from families themselves seeking to address peer needs unmet by the traditional system (Mantel et al. 1976). Mutual experiences shared in the group can minimize feelings of depression, isolation, and alienation as one learns that others have similar feelings and reactions to the illness. The support group setting creates a therapeutic structure to reinforce early constructive attitudes and improve problem-solving patterns of behavior (Johnson and Norby 1981). Perhaps the greatest advantage lies in the fact that through the group process one helps oneself, and also enjoys the satisfaction of helping others (Kaplan 1981). Families of a person recently diagnosed with cancer can gain information and skills from experienced families who can help them cope. Staff must remember that peer support groups have limitations; not all patients are comfortable in a group situation, or even in interacting with other patients. One must be aware of this and be prepared to offer to some patients less threatening ways of receiving mutual support, such as individual peer contact or individual therapy with a professional.

Groups can be defined to be many things. There can be groups for patients; there can be groups for families; there can be groups for the significant key other; and there can be groups for children of patients to discuss some of the common issues and gain support from each other. Inevitably the interest to start a group emerges in most oncology settings at one time or another. Unfortunately in most settings, the people involved will not have access to expertise in group therapy and are left on their own. This does not mean that many places have not been extraordinarily successful and innovative with their groups without a ''group therapy person'' to direct and supervise. However, it should also be borne in mind that there are certain risks attendant on any clinical process. There are always some risks when one puts patients in a situation that potentially uncovers emotions, and such emotional responses can become multiplied by the dynamics of some group processes. Groups should not be started or run casually, but thought through and custom designed in a fashion that takes into account the training and supervision available and the nature and problems of the population being served. Members of any program aspiring to initiate groups for cancer patients should make sure that they have addressed, at a minimum, the following parameters:

1. *What are the goals of the group?* Groups may intend to accomplish various goals, for example: (a) to facilitate information sharing among patients, their families, and staff; (b) to clarify problems that patients and family encounter and to encourage sharing of program-solving skills among patients and family members; (c) to provide patients and their families with an increased sense of social support during their treatment experience; (d) to teach patients about consequences of the disease and its treatment and methods of dealing with them.

2. *Will the group be open or closed?* Will the group start and stop on specified dates or will it be ongoing? Can new members join at any time? Is there any expectation of commitment to a certain number of sessions by the participants? How long can a member continue? If the group is time limited, what happens afterward?

3. *How will patients be screened?* Is there any specific thinking on what type of patients do or do not belong in the group? Often the clinicians involved feel that some sort of global judgment is sufficient to decide who should be in a group. And such judgments by

clinicians experienced in this area and with this population may be quite accurate. However, there are further questions that must be considered: (a) What about patients with substance abuse problems? (b) What about patients with major psychiatric illness? (c) What about patients whose personality would be disruptive to the group? (d) Should various diagnoses, age groups, or stages of illness be mixed?

4. *How will the group be offered to potential members?* What will patients be told about the group? By whom? After all, the population in question is not a "psychiatric population," and may not be comfortable with or familiar with the idea of group therapy. How will it be presented and what expectations will be induced by the process of bringing patients into the group?

5. *What backup and supervision are available?* Is there a clinician (psychiatrist, for example) available to consult with in the event that a significant psychiatric symptom appears in the context of the group? Is there an opportunity for the group leaders to have ongoing supervision and review of the group process?

6. *What recordkeeping should be involved?* What records will be kept where by whom and for what purpose?

7. *What will be the nature of the group process?* For example, will the group be primarily information/education oriented, or will it encourage exploration of problems? For example, suppose a person in the group asks, "How many more treatments is my husband going to need?" Will one of the group leaders simply say, "For that type of illness, usually a course of seven treatments is given." Or will the group leader assist in finding out what the person knows, what sort of communication process the person is involved in with the physician, how that communication is going, and whether the question is symptomatic of other difficulties in the relationship with the spouse or the treatment process? Will other patients be encouraged to describe their experiences as to how many treatments are involved, or to relate their ways of getting information from the system? These options would lead to different group experiences and should be thought through.

8. *How does the group fit within the overall treatment program?* Are other staff aware of its purpose and have they had opportunities to express any concerns? Have the physicians been included in planning to facilitate their support?

A reviewing of these eight points will be a helpful exercise for anyone who is starting a group. Depending on the answers, a variety of group structures are possible; each is potentially helpful in certain ways, and each involves certain risks and liabilities. We believe these dimensions should be recorded for any group program being started.

The growing literature concerning the use of groups with cancer patients has remained largely descriptive, with few controlled studies of the effectiveness of the intervention. Group approaches (Gustafson and Whitman 1978; Kopel and Mock 1978; Wood et al. 1978) have been stated to help in a variety of fashions, including the sharing of problem-solving skills and instillation of hope (Vachon and Lyall 1976), providing medical staff with better insight into patients' needs (Corder and Anders 1974), and ventilation of emotions (Parsell and Tagliareni 1975). While there have been some objections that bringing together a group of people with advanced illness and poor prognoses might be demoralizing and have a negative impact, a number of reports to the contrary indicate that such groups actually are an important means of support (Spiegel and Yalom 1978; Spiegel 1979; Yalom and Greaves 1977).

There have been a number of assessment studies addressing the impact of the group experience. Ferlic et al. (1979) reported improved self-concept, adjustment to illness, knowledge, and openness among patients as compared with a control group. Spiegel et al. (1981) reported on the effects of a weekly support group for women with metastatic carcinoma of the breast in a one-year, randomized, prospective outcome study. The groups focused on problems of illness, including relationships. Outcome variables included mood, coping strategies, and self-esteem. Eight-six patients were tested at four-month intervals. This study provided objective evidence that such an intervention improved mood, coping, and adjustment in the group patients. It should be borne in mind that the groups were run by experienced group therapists with several years of training specifically in the process used in this study. Overall there are both growing clinical interest and increasingly sophisticated evaluation methodology in the area of group interventions. Groups fall along a spectrum from ''educational'' to ''supportive'' to ''exploratory,'' and may involve knowledgeable professionals, oncology staff, nurses or social workers, or trained therapists. Whatever model is selected, this section provides parameters to consider to help reach a clearer definition of what is taking place and the resources needed to accomplish the stated goals.

Bereavement

If a patient is terminal, the final stages of life are usually spent in the hospital, or perhaps in a hospice setting, or in the patient's own house when appropriate home care programs are available. Regardless of where the patient dies, it is a natural tendency of staff who have been dealing consistently with the patient to lose contact with the family entirely. This is particularly a difficult thing for a family whose major social support network at the end tends to be the nursing staff and physicians who have been involved with the patient's care from the beginning of the illness. The abandonment that family can feel after a death can be an extremely difficult adjustment, along with the fact that they have experienced an intense personal loss. Many bereavement follow-up programs have developed whereby someone on the hospital staff who worked most closely with the family systematically makes a follow-up contact either to go over the autopsy report with the family or to ask the family whether there are any further questions about the course of the illness. At this time, it is important for the staff to make various kinds of assessments in terms of the family's adjustment. Despite occasional visits from some families to the clinic where the patient was treated, the break from the treatment team is usually a dramatic one. Staff in a hospital setting must remember that unless they make or initiate contact with the family, the family can be lost to the treatment team completely.

There are a variety of assumptions about the bereavement process that have not been investigated fully because of the inherent difficulties of this type of research, such as obtaining adequate prospective data. In a review of current cancer research compiled by the U.S. Department of Health and Human Services, none of the 27 projects listed in the area of psychosocial factors in cancer treatment look at the significant support person or at the effect of prebereavement counseling on such persons.

Approximately two million persons in the United States die each year, and of this number approximately 400,000 die from cancer. Most of these deceased persons have spouses and other close relatives who must confront the grief associated with bereavement. The general process of "uncomplicated" or normal bereavement has been described by Lindemann (1944), Parkes (1972), Marris (1958), and Kübler-Ross (1969), and has been summarized by Lazare (1979) as including an initial phase of disbelief and denial, followed by outbursts of tearfulness and restlessness alternating with numbness and blunted affect. After this phase, which may last from a few hours to several weeks, a variety of somatic symptoms often appear, including tightness in the throat and shortness of breath, along with psychological distress and preoccupation with the deceased. Then follows a review of memories associated with the deceased and discussion of the deceased with others. Eventually there is a renewal of interest in the external world. However, there is a persistence of depressive symptoms in a significant number of persons for many months.

Physical and Psychological Reactions to Bereavement

The literature regarding reactions to bereavement has been reviewed by Jacobs and Ostfeld (1977), Epstein et al. (1975), and Vachon (1976). The first systemic empirical study of bereavement was conducted in 1944 by Eric Lindemann. The reactions that he noted included psychological and somatic distress, guilt, and hostility. Other early studies also found a wide variety of negative physical and psychological reactions to bereavement. Maddison (1968) described grief reactions as including nervousness, depression, feelings of panic, nightmares, insomnia, trembling, fatigue, reduced work capacity, headaches, blurred vision, and indigestion. Parkes and Brown (1972) found that bereaved persons relative to control subjects showed greater sleep disturbances, appetite and weight fluctuations, loneliness, restlessness, and indecisiveness; poorer memory; and increased consumption of tranquilizers, alcohol, and tobacco.

Maddison and Viola (1968) found that 32% of the widows as contrasted to only 2% of the control subjects showed marked deterioration in health 13 months after bereavement. Glick et al. (1974) found that within eight weeks after bereavement, 40% of the widows had consulted their physicians because of headaches, dizziness, muscular aches, menstrual irregularities, loss of appetite, and insomnia. Maddison (1968) also noted an increase in the number of physician visits in the first year of bereavement, and Gerber et al. (1975) found a similar increase for widows with a poor prior medical history.

Greenblatt (1978) reported that physical disease, hospitalization, and mortality in widows all exceeded expected rates. Kraus and Lilienfeld (1959) and Parkes et al. (1969) found a 40% increase in mortality rates in the first six months following bereavement. Young et al. (1963) found higher relative risk of mortality for men during the first six months following bereavement, but found little differential thereafter. Cox and Ford (1964) compared death certificates and found that the mortality in widows was higher than usual in the second year of widowhood, and Rees and Lutkins (1967), in the largest and most definite cohort study, found that bereaved close relatives experienced a 12% increase in mortality during the first year of bereavement, and that the risk was greatest for widows. Some writers have found a higher incidence of mental illness requiring hospitalization among widowed than among married persons. More recently, Clayton and Darvish (1979) verified that bereavement is associated with the full range of depressive symptoms, and that although the somatic symptoms of depression tend to improve by the 13th month following bereavement, the psychological symptoms tend to persist even after this length of time. However, Heyman and Gianturco (1973) found little difference when comparing measures before and after bereavement regarding health, interests, or psychological morbidity, except for a small increase in depression. But their subjects all were elderly persons (average age, 74) and other studies have also suggested that older persons, at least older widows (Helsing and Szklo 1981) may experience less pronounced reactions to bereavement than do younger persons (Clayton 1979).

That bereavement is a process that varies over time rather than a constant state or condition has been verified by several studies that have noted varying reactions to bereavement after different periods of time following bereavement. For example, Clayton (1974) found that 35% of the bereaved subjects met the criteria for depression at four months and only 17% did so after one year. Thus, in any study of bereavement, it is important to assess the effects of bereavement at several points in time following bereavement.

Pre- and Postbereavement Psychosocial Interventions

Traditionally the family has provided support in whatever style characterizes the interaction of the particular family. For those without clearly identified support, professionals such as social workers have provided intermittent support on a costly basis. It is sometimes overlooked that well meaning family members, even when available, may not know how or have great difficulty providing support to a dying person, or in feeling supported themselves in the process. By shifting part of the focus to the supporter instead of exclusively on the patient, terminal care acknowledges the importance of a functional support network to the quality, and perhaps duration, or survival of the patient. *In addition, counseling the supporter may provide a preventive intervention for the person in the bereaved state that follows.* In her significant book, Ruth Abrams (1974) has stated: "I believe, therefore, that the goal of treatment, especially when the diseases becomes hopeless, should be not only to provide optimum care to the patient but also to recognize when those caring for him need support and comfort." Prevention is an important and underdeveloped area. It is important to clarify the process and to assess the effects of psychosocial interventions on those who are at risk for the various psychological and physical reactions to bereavement. Several studies have assessed the effects of *postbereavement* interventions on the course of reactions to bereavement. Raphael (1977) studied the effects of a postbereavement intervention in lowering morbidity during the first three months following bereavement in subjects selected as at high risk for postbereavement morbidity. Her intervention provided specific support for grief and encouragement of mourning. All subjects were followed up at 13 months postbereavement with a validated health questionnaire. There was a significant lowering of morbidity in the intervention group as compared with the control group. The most significant impact of intervention occurred with the subgroup of subjects who perceived their social networks as very nonsupportive during the bereavement crisis.

Gerber et al. (1975) studied the effects of an intervention program in which the treatment group received psychosocial support from either a psychiatric social worker or a psychiatric nurse on a variety of health measures (e.g., office visits to physicians, major illnesses, minor illnesses, use of prescriptions). Their results suggested that this intervention was successful to some extent, but that it did not have positive effects until approximately three months after the intervention was begun.

Vachon et al. (1980) compared the postbereavement adaptation of widows who had received emotional support and practical assistance from another widow with that of a control group of widows who had not received this support. They found that the adaptation of the widows who had received the support was similar to that of those who had not, but that the rate of adaptation was accelerated for the group who received the support. The subjects in this study were tested at six-, 12-, and 24-month intervals following bereavement. A follow-up of the sample at two years (Vachon et al. 1982) found that those who continued with high distress had multiple indicators of distress present and identifiable as soon as one month after bereavement. A risk factor for continued distress was dissatisfaction with available social support. Further, a short final illness of the husband was also an associated risk factor, perhaps indicating that the absence of an opportunity for anticipatory grieving may lengthen the course of grief resolution (Jacobs and Douglas 1979).

Most studies of bereavement have relied for data on the retrospective recall by the bereaved person of events and conditions prior to the death of the deceased person. Because such retrospective reports are subject to distortions, it would be preferable to obtain these data at the time of the event or condition in question, that is, prior to the death, if they pertain to events and conditions prior to the death.

Despite the number of cited studies on bereavement, only one appears to have given careful attention to the effects of the specific cause of death on the bereavement process. These authors (Vachon et al. 1977) found that the bereavement process was more difficult for widows whose husbands had died from cancer than for widows whose husbands had died from other causes, especially cardiovascular diseases. For example, they found that more widows of cancer patients than of patients with other illnesses perceived themselves to be in poor health and experienced nightmares during the initial bereavement period. Thus it appears important to control for the cause of death in studies of the course of bereavement.

No study to date appears to have investigated the effects of a *prebereavement* intervention on bereavement reactions, even though 81% of the widows in the Vachon et al. (1977) study rated the period of final illness as extremely or very stressful. Some of them felt they "could have benefited considerably from some type of counseling during the final illness—even more than from service following bereavement." It appears important, therefore, to explore the effects of a prebereavement intervention on reactions to bereavement, especially in those who may be at higher risk for bereavement associated morbidity. Thus pre- and postbereavement data can be compared.

Conclusions

Many issues face cancer patients and their families—issues that would require volumes to discuss. In this chapter, we attempted to look at some of the problems that patients and families experience related to loss of control when the diagnosis of cancer is made for a family member. The chapter also looks at the psychosocial aspects of physical disability, both acute and chronic, and some of the issues that staff can be aware of to increase the patient's ability to cope in a difficult situation. The importance of social support is historically considered, as well as its implication on the family and the impact it has on the patient with cancer. A critical component of this chapter is the role of the significant key other or spouse in the care and psychological adjustment of the patient and the entire family faced with a chronic illness. Finally, the need for the development of such interventions in the hospital and community is discussed. The following section of this book provides an expanded knowledge base of some of the medical aspects that cancer patients face and provides a critical component of the total care where a diagnosis of cancer has been made.

References

Abrams, R.: The patient with cancer—His changing pattern of communication. *N. Engl. J. Med.* 274 (1966): 317–322.

Abrams, R.: *Not alone with cancer.* Springfield, Ill.: Charles C Thomas, 1974.

Andrews, G., Tennant, C., Hewson, D. M., et al.: Life event stress, social support, coping style and risk of psychological impairment. *J. Nerv. Ment. Dis.* 166 (1978): 307–316.

Berkman, L. F.: Psychosocial resources health behavior and mortality: A nine year follow-up study. Read before APHA, October 31, 1977.

Blumberg, B. D., and Flaherty, M.: Services available to persons with cancer. *JAMA* 244 (1980): 1715–1717.

Brown, G. W., Bhrolchain, H., and Harris, T.: Social class and psychiatric disturbance among women in an urban population. *Sociology* 9 (1975): 225–254.

CANCER INFORMATION CLEARING HOUSE, NATIONAL CANCER INSTITUTE: *Coping with cancer. An annotated bibliography of public, patient, and professional information and education materials.* NIH Pub. no. 80-2129, 1980.

_____: *Coping with cancer. A resource for the health professional.* NIH Pub. no. 80-2080, 1980.

_____: *Taking time. Support for people with cancer and the people who care about them.* NIH Pub. no. 81-2059, 1981.

CAPONE, M. A., GOOD, R. S., WESTIE, K. S., AND HACOBSON, A. F.: Psychosocial rehabilitation of gynecologic oncology patients. *Arch. Phys. Med. Rehab.* 61 (1980): 128-132.

CASSEL, J.,: Social science in epidemiology: Psychosocial processes and "stress" theoretical formulation. *Int. J. Health Serv.* 4 (1974), 3: 471-482.

CLAYTON, P. J.: Mortality and morbidity in the first year of widowhood. *Arch. Gen. Psychiatry* 30 (1974): 747-750.

_____: The sequelae and nonsequelae of conjugal bereavement. *Am. J. Psychiatry* 136 (1979): 1530-1534.

CLAYTON, P. J., AND DARVISH, J. H. S.: Course of depressive symptoms following the stress of bereavement. In J. Barrett, R. M. Rose, and G. L. Klerman (Eds.), *Stress and mental disorder.* New York: Raven Press, 1979.

COBB, S.: A model for life events and their consequences. In B. S. Dohrenwend and B. Dohrenwend (Eds.), *Stressful life events.* New York: Wiley 1974.

COBB, S.: Social support as a moderator of life stress. *Psychosom. Med.* 38 (1976): 300-312.

CORDER, M. P., AND ANDERS, R. L.: Death and dying: Oncology discussion group. *JPN Ment. Health Soc.* 12 (1974): 10-14.

COX, P. R., AND FORD, J. R.: The mortality of widows shortly after widowhood. *Lancet* 1 (1964): 163-164.

CRAIG, T. J., AND ABELOFF, M. D.: Psychiatric symptomatology among hospitalized cancer patients. *Am. J. Psychiatry* 131 (1974): 1323-1327.

CROMES, G. F., JR.: Implementation of interdisciplinary cancer rehabilitation. *Rehab. Counseling Bull.* 21 (1978): 230-237.

DEMPSEY, G. M., BUCHSBAUM, H. J., AND MORRISON, J.: Psychosocial adjustment to pelvic extenteration. *Gyneiol. Oniol.* 3 (1975): 325-334.

DEROGATIS, L. R., AND KOURLESIS, S. M.: An approach to evaluation of sexual problems in the cancer patient. *CA-Cancer J. Clin.* 31 (1981): 46-50.

DEVLIN, H. B., PLANT, J. A., AND GRIFFIN, M.: Aftermath of surgery for anorectal cancer. *Br. Med. J.* 3 (1971): 413–418.

DIETZ H: Cancer: the medical factors in J. Garrett and E. S. Levine (Eds.), *Rehabilitation factors in the physically disabled.* New York: Columbia University Press, pp. 149–208.

DOHRENWEND, B. S. AND DOHRENWEND, B. P.: Life stress and illness: Formulation of the issues. In B. S. Dohrenwend and B. P. Dohrenwend (Eds.), *Stressful life events and their contexts.* New York: Prodist, 1981, pp. 1–27.

DONAHUE, V. C., AND KNAPP, R. C.: Sexual rehabilitation of gynecologic cancer patients. *Obstet. Gynecol.* 49 (1977): 118–121.

DURKHEIM, E.: *Suicide.* New York: Free Press, 1951.

EPSTEIN, G., WEITZ, L., ROBACK, H., AND McKEE, E.: Research on bereavement: A selective and critical review. *Compr. Psychiatry* 16 (1975): 537–546.

FERLIC, M., GOLDMAN, A., AND KENNEDY, B. J.: Group counseling in adult patients with advanced cancer. *Cancer* 43 (1979): 760–766.

FIEFEL, H.: *New meaning of death.* New York: McGraw-Hill, 1977.

FORESTER, B., KORNFELD, D. S., AND FLEISS, J.: Effects of psychotherapy on patient distress during radiotherapy for cancer. *Psychosom. Med.* 44 (1982): 118.

FREIDENBERGS, I., ET AL.: Psychological aspects of cancer: Annotated bibliography. *JSAS Catalog of Selected Documents in Psychology* 9 (1979): 61 (Ms. No. 1890).

FRENCH, J. R. P., JR., RODGERS, W., AND COBB, S.: Adjustment as person-environment fit. In G. V. Coelho, D. A. Hamburg, and J. E. Adams (Eds.), *Coping and adaptation.* New York: Basic Books, 1974.

GERBER, I., WIENER, A., BATTIN, D., AND ARKIN, A. M.: Brief therapy to the aged bereaved. In Schoenberg, et al. (Eds.), *Bereavement: Its psychosocial aspects.* New York: Columbia University Press, 1975.

GERLE, B., LUNDIN, G., AND SANDBLOM, P.: The patient with inoperable cancer from the psychiatric and social standpoint. *Cancer* 13 (1960): 1206–1217.

GLICK, I. O., WEISS, R. S., AND PARKES, C. M.: *The first year of bereavement.* New York: Wiley, 1974.

GOLDBERG, R. J., AND WOOL, M.: "Social support and adaptation in cancer patients. Description of counseling intervention with the 'significant key other'." 1982, unpublished manuscript.

GORDON, W. A., FREIDENBERGS, I., DILLER, L., HIBBARD, M., WOLF, C., LEVINE, L., LIPKINS, R., EZRACHI, O., AND LUCIDO, D.: Efficacy of psychosocial intervention with cancer patients. *J. Consult. Clin. Psychol.* 48 (1980): 743–759.

GOTTESMAN, D., AND LEWIS, M. S.: Differences in crisis reactions among cancer and surgery patients. *J. Consult. Clin. Psychol.* 50 (1982): 381–388.

GREENBLATT, M.: The grieving spouse. *Am. J. Psychiatry* 135 (1978): 43–47.

GUSTAFSON, J., AND WHITMAN, H.: Towards a balanced social environment on the oncology service. *Soc. Psychiatry* 13 (1978): 147–152.

HACKETT, T. P.: Psychological assistance for the dying patient and his family. *Ann. Rev. Med.* (1976): 371–378.

HARVEY, R. F., HOLLIS, M. J., AND HABECK, R. V.: Cancer rehabilitation; An analysis of 36 program approaches. *JAMA* 247 (1982): 2127–2131.

HELLER, K.: The effects of social support: Prevention and treatment implications. In A. P. Goldstein and F. H. Kanfer (Eds.), *Maximizing treatment gains: Transfer enhancement in psychotherapy.* New York: Academic Press, 1978.

HELSING, K. J., AND SZKLO, M.: Mortality after bereavement. *Am. J. Epidemiol.* 114 (1981): 41–52.

HEYMAN, K. D., AND GIANTURCO, D. T.: Long-term adaptation by the elderly to bereavement. *J. Gerontol.* 28 (1973): 359–362.

JACOBS, S., AND DOUGLAS, L.: Grief: A mediating process between a loss and illness. *Compr. Psychiatry* 20 (1979): 165–176.

JACOBS, S., AND OSTFELD, A.: An epidemiological review of the mortality of bereavement. *Psychosom. Med.* 39 (1977): 344–357.

JARVIS, J. H.: Post-mastectomy breast phantoms. *J. Nerv. Ment. Dis.* 144 (1967): 266–272.

JEWETT, H. J.: The present status of radical prostatectomy for stages A and B prostatic cancer. *Urol. Clin. N. Am.* 2 (1975): 105–124.

JOHNSON, J. L., AND NORBY, P.: we can, we can: A program for cancer families. *Cancer Nurs.* 4 (1981): 1–23.

KAPLAN, ANNE: Social support: A construct and its measurement. Senior Honors Thesis, Brown University, May 1977.

KAPLAN, D. M., SMITH, A., GROBSTEIN, R., AND FISCHMAN, S. E.: Family mediation of stress. *Soc. Work* 18 (1973): 60–69.

KAPLAN, G.: The mastery of stress: Psychologic aspects. *Am. J. Psychiatry* 138 (1981): 413–420.

KAPLAN, R. H., CASSEL, J. C., AND GORE, S.: Social support and health. *Med. Care* 15 (1977), (5): 471–482, supplement.

KASTENBAUM, R., AND AISENBURG, R.: *The psychology of death.* New York: Springer, 1976.

KOPEL, K., AND MOCK, L.A.: The use of group sessions for the emotional support of families of terminal patients. *Death Educ.* 1 (1978): 409–422.

Krant, M. J., and Johnston, L.: Family members' perceptions of communications in late stage cancer. *Int. J. Psychiatr. Med.* 8 (1977–1978): 203–216.

Kraus, A. S., and Lilienfeld, A. M.: Some epidemiological aspects of the high mortality rate in the young widowed group. *J. Chronic Dis.* 10 (1959): 207.

Kubler-Ross, E.: *On death and dying.* New York: Macmillan, 1969.

Lazare, A.: Unresolved grief. In A. Lazare (Ed.), *Outpatient psychiatry.* Baltimore: Williams & Wilkins, 1979.

Lindemann, E.: Symptomatology and management of acute grief. *Am. J. Psychiatry* 101 (1944): 141–148.

Linn, M. W., Linn, B. S., and Harris, R.: Effects of counseling for late stage cancer patients. *Cancer* 49 (1982): 1048–1055.

Maddison, D.: The relevance of conjugal bereavement for preventive psychiatry. *Br. J. Med. Psychol.* 41 (1968): 223–233.

Maddison, D., and Raphael, B.: The family of the dying patient. In B. Schoenberg, A. C. Carr, D. Peretz, and A. H. Kutscher (Eds.), *Psychosocial aspects of terminal care.* New York: Columbia University Press, 1972, pp. 185–200.

Maddison, D., and Viola, A.: The health of widows in the year following bereavement. *J. Psychosom. Res.* 12 (1968): 297.

Maguire, G. P. et al.: Psychiatric problems in the first year after mastectomy. *Br. Med. J.* 1 (1978): 963–965.

Mantel, J., Alexander, E., and Kleinman, M.: Social work with self-help groups. *Health Soc. Work* 1 (1976): 86–100.

Marris, P.: *Widows and their families.* London: Routledge & Kegan Paul, 1958.

McAleer, C. A., and Kluge, C. A.: Why cancer rehabilitation? *Rehab. Couns. Bull.* 21 (1978): 208–215.

Mechanic, D.: Social structure and personal adaptation: Some neglected dimensions. In C. V. Coelho, D. A. Hamburg, and J. E. Adams (Eds.), *Coping and adaptation.* New York: Basic Books, 1974, pp. 32–44.

Miller, C., Denner, P., and Richardson, V.: Assisting the psychosocial problems of cancer patients: A review of current research. *Int. J. Nurs. Stud.* 13 (1976): 161–166.

Mitchell, J. C. (Ed.): *Social networks in urban situations.* Manchester: University Press, 1969.

Morris, T., Greer, H. S., and White, P. W.: Psychological and social adjustment to mastectomy. *Cancer* 40 (1977): 2381–2387.

OLSEN, E. H.: The impact of serious illness in the family system. *Postgrad. Med.* 47 (1970): 169–174.

PARKES, C. M.: *Bereavement: Studies of grief in adult life.* New York: International Universities Press, 1972.

PARKES, C. M., BENJAMIN, B., AND FITZGERALD, R. G.: Broken heart: a statistical study of increased mortality among widowers. *Br. Med. J.* 1 (1969): 740.

PARKES, C. M., AND BROWN, R. J.: Health after bereavement: A controlled study of young Boston widows and widowers. *Psychosom. Med.* 34 (1972): 449–461.

PARSELL, S., AND TAGLIARENI, E. M.: Cancer patients help each other. *Am. J. Nurs.* 74 (1975): 650–651.

PECK, A.: Emotional reactions to having cancer. *J. Roentgenol. Rad. Ther. Nucl. Med.* 114 (1972): 591–599.

PETEET, J. R.: A closer look at the concept of support: Some applications to the care of patients with cancer. *Gen. Hosp. Psychiatr.* 4 (1982): 19–23.

PLUMB, M. M., AND HOLLAND, J.: Comparative studies of psychological function in patients with advanced cancer II: Interviewer rated current and past psychological symptoms. *Psychosom. Med.* 43 (1981): 243–254.

RAPHAEL, B.: Preventive intervention with the recently bereaved. *Arch. Gen. Psychiatry* 34 (1977): 1450–1454.

REES, W. D., AND LUTKINS, S. G.: Mortality of bereavement. *Br. Med. J.* 4 (1967): 13–16.

ROTMAN, M., ROGOW, L., DeLEON, G., AND HESKEL, N.: Supportive therapy in radiation oncology. *Cancer* 39 (1977): 744–750.

SCHAIN, W.: Psychological impact of the diagnosis of breast cancer on the patient. *Front. Rad. Ther. Onc.* 11: 68–69, 1976.

SHNEIDMAN, E. S.: *Death: Current Perspectives.* Palo Alto, Calif.: Mayfield, 1976. Silberfarb, P. M.: Psychiatric themes in the rehabilitation of mastectomy patients. *Int. J. Psychiatr. Med.* 8 (1977–1978): 159–167.

SIMONTON, O. C., MATTHEWS-SIMONTON, S., AND SPARKS, T. F.: Psychological intervention in the treatment of cancer. *Psychosomatics* 21 (Mar. 1980): 226–233.

SPIEGEL, D.: Psychological support for women with metastatic carcinoma. *Psychosomatics* 20 (1979): 780–787.

SPIEGEL, D., BLOOM, J. R., AND YALOM, I.: Group support for patients with metastatic cancer. *Arch. Gen. Psychiatr.* 38 (May 1981): 527–533.

Spiegel, D., and Yalom, I. D.: A support group for dying patients. *Int. J. Group Psychother.* 28 (1978): 233–245.

Turner, R. J.: Social support as a contingency in psychological well-being. *J. Health Soc. Behav.* 22 (1981): 357–367.

Vachon, M. L. S.: Grief and bereavement following the death of a spouse. *Can. Psychiatr. Assoc. J.* 21 (1976): 35–44.

Vachon, M. L., and Lyall, W. A.: Applying psychiatric techniques to patients with cancer. *Hosp. Commun. Psychiatry* 27 (1976): 582–584.

Vachon, M. L. S., Freedman, K., Formo, A., Rogers, J., Lyall, W. A. L., and Freeman, S. J. J.: The final illness in cancer: The widow's perspective. *CMA J.* 117 (1977): 1151–1154.

Vachon, M. L. S., Lyall, W. A. L., Rogers, J., Freedman-Letofsky, K., and Freeman, S. J. J.: A controlled study of self-help intervention for widows. *Am. J. Psychiatry* 137 (1980): 1380–1384.

Vachon, M. L. S., Rogers, J., Lyall, A., Lancee, W. J., Sheldon, A. R., and Freeman, S. J. J.: Predictors and correlates of adaptation to conjugal bereavement. *Am. J. Psychiatry* 139 (1982): 998–1002.

VonEschenbach, A. C.: Sexual dysfunction following therapy for cancer of the prostate, testis, and penis. In J. M. Vaeth, *Frontiers of radiation therapy and oncology: Proceedings of the 14th Annual San Francisco Cancer Symposium, 1979.* Basel: Karger, 1980, pp. 42–50.

Weisman, A. D.: *On dying and denying.* New York: Behavioral Publications, 1972.

Weisman, A. D., and Worden, J. W.: Psychosocial analysis of cancer deaths. *Omega* 6 (1975), 1: 61–75.

————: Psychosocial screening and intervention with cancer patients: *Research report.* CA-19797, 1977–1980, 1980.

Wellisch, D. K., Jamison, K. R., and Pasnau, R. O.: Psychosocial aspects of mastectomy: II. The man's perspective. *Am. J. Psychiatry* 135 (1978): 543–546.

Wood, P. E., Milligan, I., Christ, D. et al.: Group counseling for cancer patients in a community hospital. *Psychosomatics* 19: 555–561, 1978.

Worden, J. W., and Weisman, A. D.: Do cancer patients really want counseling? *Gen. Hosp. Psychiatry* 2 (1980): 100–103.

Yalom, I. D., and Greaves, C.: Group therapy with the terminally ill. *Am. J. Psychiatry* 134 (1977): 396–400.

Young, M., Benjamin, B. and Wallis, C.: The mortality of widows. *Lancet* 2 (1963): 454–456.

PART II

Behavioral Changes in Cancer Patients

CHAPTER 4

Medical Disorders Masquerading as Psychiatric Symptoms

**Organic Mental Disorders and the
Biological Dimension of Depression**

THOUGH EXPERIENCE OF A MAJOR medical illness can be very stressful and disruptive, altered mood or behavior in cancer patients should not automatically be labeled a "psychological" reaction. Biologic impairment of brain function can produce conditions which, on the surface, appear indistinguishable from a wide variety of psychological disorders. The development of a systematic approach to psychosocial problems in cancer patients has been hampered by the scientifically unsupported view that psychological distress such as depression is an inevitable aspect of the disease. For example, "Wouldn't you be depressed if you had cancer?" frequently functions as a disclaimer for closer evaluation of the problem. However, any psychiatric symptom should be regarded as analogous to fever, jaundice, or anemia, which requires differential diagnostic evaluation. The purpose of this chapter is to present information about commonly encountered biologic factors

83

that contribute to patient disabilities that are often mistakenly presumed to be "psychogenic."

Organic Mental Disorders (OMD) in Cancer Patients

Since complex medical problems are so prevalent in patients with cancer, organically induced mental disorders *should be the first consideration in the evaluation of any medical patient who develops impaired mood, thought, or behavior.* This section reviews the wide variety of medical disorders that can lead to impairment of neural function in the central nervous system (CNS), which is the final common denominator in all OMDs. The symptoms that result from CNS impairment depend on the region and severity of the insult. Generalized metabolic impairment often leads to delirium, referred to by Engel (1959) as a "syndrome of cerebral insufficiency." Delirium, which often fluctuates in its clinical course, is characterized by:

1. Difficulty in sustaining attention.
2. Disorientation and memory impairment.
3. Perceptual distortion (along a continuum from misperceptions to hallucinations).
4. Increased or decreased psychomotor activity.
5. Insomnia or daytime drowsiness.

In its most dramatic form, delirium is easily recognized since the patient is obviously confused and agitated, and may have frightening or disturbing sensory distortions. In less severe cases, OMD may be recognized only by challenging the person with specific mental status questions (Folstein and McHugh 1975) since many patients mask their confusion by appearing to be quiet, depressed, or anxious. Behavioral changes in medical patients often are the outcome of underlying cognitive impairment.

Jane R. is a 52-year-old married mother of two children who had assisted her husband in his insurance business until two years ago when she was diagnosed with carcinoma of the breast. Following a mastectomy and radiation treatment, she did well for approximately one year, when she began to develop some change in her personality. She became more irritable at home and short tempered with her family and friends. It became uncomfortable for people to be around her and everyone began to wonder what was going on with this formerly pleasant and sociable woman who had no previous history of nervous disorders. Various hypotheses were suggested by the friends and family. Some thought that the one-year anniversary of her breast surgery brought back painful feelings that were influencing her behavior. Others felt that she was "keeping too much inside" and was refusing to confront the serious nature of her illness. Still others speculated that she was purposely driving people away to ease the emotional pain for everyone involved. Amid all the speculation about her personality change, the patient suddenly developed a seizure disorder, was admitted to the hospital, and was diagnosed as having a brain tumor metastatic from her original breast cancer. In retrospect, the location of this tumor had probably accounted for her personality change all along. Personality or behavior change is not an unusual initial presentation of tumor involvement of the brain (Posner 1971). The patient was treated with further irradiation and placed on steroids to control brain swelling. About one week after starting on steroids, her personality underwent another remarkable shift—she became phenomenally energetic, euphoric, and talkative. The family was encouraged by this remarkable change in her outlook and felt that she must have been feeling very encouraged by the successful management of her symptoms. However, within a few days her speech became more inappropriate and somewhat incoherent; she began to describe frightening apparitions in her room. At this point, the family felt the emotional strain had "driven her crazy," though her doctor recognized that this woman was having psychotic symptoms as a direct secondary result of steroid treatment. The addition of another medication, haloperidol (Haldol), resulted in normalization of her mood and speech, and disappearance of hallucinations. Such effects of steroids regularly occur in a small percentage of patients and are not unique to this case (Carroll 1977; Ling et al. 1981). Aside from euphoria or psychosis, steroids can produce symptoms of depression, which can be a source of confusion for both the patient and physician. Psychiatric symptoms can occur when the steroid dose is being raised, when it is being maintained, or when it is being tapered off. It is commonly implicated in psychiatric symptoms that develop concurrently with its use, though it is not often easy to sort out the relative contribution of the steroid from the underlying medical condition.

Recognition of brain impairment resulting in an organic mental disorder is important because it often has a specific cause and treatment; failure to treat may lead to permanent deficits and unnecessary suffering. It has been estimated that 33% of hospitalized medical patients have serious cognitive impairment (Knights and Folstein 1977), and that delirium is frequently misdiagnosed as a behavioral problem (Levine et al. 1978). A recent collaborative study of the prevalence of psychiatric disorders among cancer patients found 8% to have organic mental disorders (Derogatis et al. 1983). A number of studies have documented that a large number of patients with presumed psychiatric disorders actually have medical illnesses that either directly cause or greatly exacerbate their symptoms (Hall et al. 1978; Hoffman 1982; Koranyi 1979).

> Ronald S. is a 62-year-old electrician who has been in treatment for three years for multiple myeloma. He was able to maintain his job over that time by working intermittently, though he finally decided at age 62 to begin his retirement. Within six months of his retirement, the patient's family noted a significant change in his personality, style of interaction with other people, and level of function at home. He became increasingly reclusive and inhospitable to visitors. He gave up his usual hobbies and uncharacteristically left things in disarray around the house. As in the previous case, his wife and acquaintances easily found sufficient reason to explain his change in behavior. They felt he was suffering from a "retirement syndrome." Frustrated by increasing difficulty, his wife convinced him to see his physician for counseling. Before considering referral for "retirement counseling," the physician ordered routine metabolic screening, which revealed that the patient had an excessive calcium level. An elevated calcium level (known as hypercalcemia) is the most frequent metabolic consequence of being host to a malignant disease (Segaloff 1981). It is now recognized that hypercalcemia is frequently associated with a variety of psychiatric symptoms, including psychotic features, depression, and anxiety (Weizman et al. 1979). Upon careful questioning, the patient revealed for the first time that he felt significantly depressed and was having strange and frightening hallucinatory experiences. He explained that some of his sudden unexplained departures from home were actually an attempt to flee from fearful visions. Following admission to the hospital and correction of the excess calcium level, he reported a termination of his psychotic expe-

riences and began to relate to his family in a much more typical fashion.

As another example:

Mrs. L is a 58-year-old wife of a restaurateur who, with two grown children living near her, had to be admitted to the hospital for a biopsy of a lung tumor, which was discovered on a routine chest X-ray. Her health was otherwise fine, and to no one's surprise she appeared quite well following the procedure, despite the fact that she had received general anesthesia. She was very talkative, perhaps a bit more so than her usual self, a factor that the family attributed to some anxiety and her need to reassure everyone that she was fine. The first hint of something amiss was noted by her son, who felt that she was using profanities more openly than he had ever heard, even though they were in an appropriate context, referring to people she disliked. Soon the entire family began to feel uncomfortable about her apparent lack of propriety—her language became an embarrassment, though the patient herself did not seem aware of any problem. Since the problem did not just go away by ignoring it, the family began to fear that mother was "losing her mind" because of the strain of her fears over possibly having lung cancer. Reluctantly, they called in a psychiatric consultant. By carefully reviewing her operative record, it was determined that the patient had experienced a transient, though significant, fall in her blood pressure during the biopsy procedure. This drop in blood pressure had deprived the brain of required levels of blood supply and oxygen for a period of time long enough to cause some generalized damage to her brain cells. There is some suspicion that strokes secondary to transient lowering of blood pressure are more common in the elderly than generally realized (Mitchinson 1980). Inappropriate social behavior is not an uncommon outcome when there is impairment of the function of the frontal areas of the brain. The patient was not crazy and she and the family were told that most likely her normal behavior would gradually return over the following weeks. They found this information reassuring and were able to manage until recovery did occur about two months later.

Changes of a psychological nature are not uncommon following general anesthesia. Their incidence increases with the age of the patient and the duration of anesthesia. Older brains have an increased vulnerability to physical insults of all sorts and do not have the "reserve" to withstand the fluctuations in metabolic support that may occur with major surgery. Fortunately, many of the changes gradually improve with time, though everyone knows of people who are just "never the same again" after a major operation.

The clinician should be suspicious of the presence of an organic basis to a change in mood or behavior, especially if that change occurs suddenly. Those providers who get to know the patient well, or speak with family members, are in a better position to be aware of changes in the baseline function of the patient. Nurses or social workers may need to bring such changes to the attention of the consulting physician, since he/she may not be as aware of the patient's baseline status.

Symptoms that should raise questions about an underlying organic disorder include:

Mood
Depressive symptoms
Inappropriate euphoria
Sudden extreme fluctuations
Sudden onset of crying for no apparent reason
Marked anxiety
Thought
Memory difficulties
Disorientation
Intellectual difficulties
A problem with thinking of the names of things
Confusion
Changes in level of awareness
Personality/behavior
Poor or questionable judgment
Inappropriate behavior
Withdrawal
Uncooperativeness
Irritability
Aggressiveness or hostility
Suspiciousness

The following section lists a number of impairments, commonly occuring in cancer patients, which are often overlooked when they are present as a "psychiatric" symptom (see Table 4-1).

TABLE 4.1

Causes of Organic Mental Disorders in Cancer Patients

Cause	Disorder
Metabolic	Abnormalities in glucose, BUN, sodium, potassium, hepatic function, magnesium, calcium, thyroid function, parathyroid function, oxygenation, cortisol metabolism
Electrical	Seizures and postictal states
Neoplastic	Primary brain tumors; brain metastases
Mechanical	CNS bleeding; hydrocephalus; subdural hematomas
Infectious	Meningoencephalitis, multifocal leukoencephalopathy
Drug	See Table 5.1
Arterial	Nonbacterial thrombotic endocarditis; other thromboembolic or ischemic infarcts
Degenerative	''Remote'' effects of carcinoma
Nutritional	B_{12}, folate, thiamine deficiency

Metabolic encephalopathy (brain impairment) is the single most common neurologic complication in the hospitalized cancer patients (Posner 1971) and accounts for a significant number of problems misdiagnosed as being psychiatric. The most common metabolic consequence of being host to a malignant disease is *hypercalcemia* (Segaloff 1981). Hypercalcemia most frequently presents in breast cancer patients, though it also occurs in association with bronchogenic carcinoma and other malignancies. In addition to the current interest in the medical dimensions of this disorder (Ralston et al. 1982; Sherwood 1980; Stewart et al. 1980; Wong and Freier 1982), the psychiatric implications of hypercalcemia are significant. In one study of 12 cancer patients with hypercalcemia, seven were found to have psychiatric symptoms including depression, anxiety, paranoid psychosis, and delirium (Weizman et al. 1979). *Liver failure* frequently complicates any cancer that metastasizes to that organ and results in changes in brain functions (Shafer and Jones 1982) that can produce fluctuating confusion, restlessness, and emotional lability. *Hyponatremia* (low sodium) can result from tumors such as carcinoma of the lung, which produce the syndrome of inappropriate secretion of antidiuretic hormone (SIADH). In addition to neurologic symptoms such as headache, increased intracranial pressure, ataxia (loss of balance), and seizures, low sodium can lead to cognitive impairment and confusion that may affect behavior and mood, though primary mood disturbance *per se* has not been attributed to this abnormality (Gehi et al. 1981). Vomiting or diarrhea, as well as long-term diuretic therapy, can lead to hypomagnesemia (low magnesium levels). Psychiatric symptoms may be the first manifestation of magnesium imbalance and may persist for several days after the magnesium level has returned to normal (Webb and Gehi 1981). Symptoms include personality change, nervousness, irritability, and restlessness. Depression can be a later sequelum (Hall and Joffe 1973). When a patient with pulmonary impairment exhibits any sudden change in mood, thought, or behavior, the clinician should have blood gases checked to determine whether or not there has been a significant decrease in the patient's oxygen level. *Endocrine imbalances*, including hypothyroidism and disturbances in cortisol metabolism (Carroll 1977; Ling et al. 1981) may be responsible for depressive symptoms. Carcinoid tumors produce permanent psychiatric symptoms such as depression, anxiety, or confusion about 40% of the time (Thorson et al. 1958). In addition, a series of ectopically produced psychoactive hormonal substances, including parathormone, vasopressin, methionine enkephalin (Pullan et al. 1980), and beta-endorphin and ACTH (Anderson and McHugh 1971), are increasingly being recognized as possibly responsible for mental status changes in some patients. As high as 16% of patients with lung tumors may have nonmetastatic cerebral effects (Croft and Wilkinson 1965). Such neuroendocrine factors have been hypothesized to account for depressive symptoms associated with pancreatic cancer (Klatchko et al. 1982).

Central nervous system tumor or metastases can present as psychiatric symptoms (Malamud 1967). Cerebral metastases commonly complicate cancer of the lung, breast, malignant melanoma, and choriocarcinoma. While few clinicians would mistake the generalized tonic-clonic activity of a grand mal seizure, the wide variety of psychiatric disturbances that can be the concomitant of seizure activity are not well appreciated. In one early study, a change in personality was noted to be the first sign of frontal lobe tumor (Strauss and Keschner 1935). In another review of 68 cases of cerebral metastases, 30% had behavioral or mental changes as the presenting symptom (Posner 1971). Subjective emotional symptoms including feelings of intense depression, euphoria, paranoia, or severe anxiety with a sense of impending doom can appear with temporal lobe tumors. Anxiety is the most common emotional

state associated with a temporal lobe seizure (Weil 1959). Disturbances of intellect or affect are the first clinical symptoms in approximately 20% of patients with temporal lobe tumors (Keschner
and Bender 1936). Episodes of severe anxiety or an increase in
general anxiety levels can, of course, be directly caused by a variety of medical disorders (Goldberg 1982). In addition to tumors
involving the brain, tumors of the spinal cord at times may produce symptoms that are considered "psychiatric," as they may
create unusual changes in sensation or muscle function that can be
mis-diagnosed as "conversion reactions" (Epstein et al. 1971).
Memory deficits and even amnesia can be early symptoms of tumors of the diencephalon (brain stem), especially the floor of the
third ventricle (Hecaen and Ajuriaguerra 1956; Williams and
Pennybacker 1954).

Cancer patients also appear prone to the development of *nonbacterial thrombotic endocarditis*, which may lead to cerebral embolism
(Bryan 1969; Mackenzie and Popkin 1980). This disorder is not
rare and accounts for an estimated 10% of all cerebral embolic
events (Barron et al. 1976). Eighty percent of cases of nonbacterial
thrombotic endocarditis are associated with known or occult carcinoma, most often from the pancreas, colon, or lung (Rosen and
Armstrong 1973). According to one study, 30% of the resulting
symptoms are without focal neurologic signs (Reagan and Okazaki 1974) and present instead with abrupt onset of delirium or selective cognitive impairment. A stepwise progression of symptoms
of organic mental disorder should raise the questions of ongoing
embolization associated with this disorder. Computerized axial to-
mography (CAT) scans of the brain supplemented by electroen-
cephalograms (EEG) are the definitive diagnostic tests for cerebral
tumors, though some false negative studies may result from old
machines with low resolution.

Some lymphomas (most commonly acute lymphoblastic leukemia as well as carcinoma of the breast, lung, pancreas, stomach,
or prostate) are associated with cerebral carcinomatosis. This disorder, in which carcinoma invades the brain and its surrounding
membranes without producing bulky mass lesions, may present as
a mental disorder (Posner 1971). Obviously all patients with
changes in mood, thought, or behavior should also have a careful
neurological exam search for associated signs of CNS involvement.

The cancer patient is predisposed to CNS infections (Armstrong et al. 1971; Chernik et al. 1978) because of altered host re-

sistance, the tumor itself, the chemotherapy, and the hospital environment. A number of bacteria can be involved in addition to fungal and viral agents. While a CNS infection can present as an overwhelming medical catastrophe, at other times it may run a more subacute course with waxing and waning of symptoms of attention or behavioral disturbance. For this reason, patients with presumed psychiatric disturbances should have their temperatures checked, even if they are referred to a nonmedical clinician for a presumed psychiatric problem. Finally, there are reports of cancer causing degenerative changes in the CNS without the presence of metastases. These "remote effects" of carcinoma (Corsellis 1969; Hochberg 1981; Shapiro 1976; Yahr et al. 1965) most likely do occur, though they can usually be diagnosed only by exclusion.

Some of the side effects of *radiotherapy* can be associated with presumed or actual psychiatric consequences (Allen 1978; Goldberg et al. 1982). Early reactions occur during or immediately following radiation therapy that may be uncomfortable, though they are self-limiting. Such effects include loss of appetite, nausea and vomiting, or diarrhea, which can create a sense of debilitation having secondary depressive effects. Acute encephalopathy can occur immediately following large dose fractions. Subacutely, demyelination can follow two to three months after brain irradiation. More delayed radiation injury, related to a degree of vascular sclerosis, can develop months to years after treatment (Sheline 1980). There has been recent attempts to study the long-term effects of brain irradiation on mental functioning (Meadows et al. 1981). Long-term follow-up of children who have received prophylactic cranial irradiation has demonstrated some decreased intellectual capacity compared with children with similar disease who did not receive such irradiation (Moss et al. 1981). There have been, as yet, no documentation of intellectual impairment in adults as a result of radiation treatments.

The Psychobiology of Depression in Cancer Patients

While there have been significant strides in unraveling the underlying biology of depression, the general public, as well as some sectors of the medical community, continue to lack information regarding this disorder.

Much of the difficulty in understanding depression arises from the fact that the same word is used to describe such a variety of situations. For instance, depression is used to refer to the transient disappointments we all feel following some minor failure or loss. Such brief reactive states can hardly be considered an "illness," and it would be more accurate to refer to such situations as adjustment problems characterized by depressive features. Uncomplicated grief or bereavement can be mistakenly called depression. Again, however, the majority of people go through a process of grief that is self-limited and culturally sanctioned. Depression can be used to refer to the experience of some individuals whose personality structure is characterized by a chronically negative outlook. It also is used to describe a collection of the somatic sequelae of physical illness such as fatigue, loss of appetite, sleeping difficulty, and difficulty in concentrating. Such depressions are actually secondary to the systemic consequences of medical illness or may be associated with an organic mental disorder, as discussed in the previous section. Finally, depression can be used to describe a severe and disabling constellation of physical and psychological symptoms that appear to have an underlying biologic basis. This type of depression is now referred to by a number of terms, including primary or major depression (or affective disorder).

How many cancer patients develop a major depressive episode? Up until recently, estimates have depended on anecdotal impressions of individual clinicians. Over the past five years, an increasing clinical and research liaison between psychiatry and oncology program has begun to produce formal research data gathered in a systematic fashion. The prevalence of depression in cancer patients has been widely reported as 37% (Peck 1972), 50% (Hinton 1972), and even as high as 75% (Craig and Abeloff 1974) in hospitalized cancer patients referred to psychiatry. However, such figures are generally inflated by studies restricted to samples unrepresentative of the general population of cancer patients. Furthermore, the evaluative questionnaires used to assess depression can be misleading because many of the somatic symptoms of cancer and its treatment can inflate the overall score artificially, indicating the presence of depression when the patient actually is not suffering from the kind of pessimism and self-deprecatory thoughts that are characteristic of patients with actual depression. When one is careful to separate the psychological from the illness-related physical symptoms, it seems that about 20% of patients with advanced cancer have at least moderately severe depression (Plumb and Holland 1977; Derogatis et al. 1983). In the case of the cancer patient, a wide variety of medical complications can create symptoms that can mislead the patient and clinician into assuming that depression exists; likewise, many signs and symptoms can be mistakenly ascribed to depression that actually are a result of the medical illness (see previous section).

When symptoms associated with depression are accounted for by some underlying medical disorder, they are called "secondary depressions" to distinguish them from "primary" major depression (in which there is no such medically identifiable cause). Depression is especially difficult to diagnose in the face of pain and often disappears when pain is adequately treated. The primary treatment of all secondary depression involves correction of the underlying medical condition. It is important to be clear that such secondary depression can be clinically indistinguishable from a primary psychiatric depressive disorder. For example, in the midst of depression secondary to hypothyroidism, the patient may feel worthless and excessively guilty for past behavior, and will be able to reveal, during a psychiatric interview, a number of significant childhood and developmental events that logically could contribute to the depressive condition. In fact, it is not unusual for such patients to participate in psychotherapy for long periods of time during which both the patient and therapist are convinced that the depression has a psychological basis. However, correction of the underlying medical disorder, once it is recognized, often will result in resolution of the symptoms and a disappearance of the negative preoccupation with past events formerly seen as so disturbing. This discussion does not imply that patients with medically based depressive symptoms require only medical treatment to the exclusion of consideration of their emotional and personal concerns (Goldberg 1981). Whatever the underlying cause of depressive symptoms, the experience of the patient must be considered. If a person with depressive symptoms of fatigue and poor concentration secondary to potassium deficiency, for example, is not "truly" depressed to begin with, he or she most likely will develop decreased self-esteem and impaired interpersonal relationships if the symptoms remain untreated long enough.

Consider the following example of a patient whose depressive symptoms were mistakenly ascribed to psychogenic causes:

> Edwin R. is a 47-year-old accountant who is married and is the father of three children. He had been in good health his entire life until one morning he awoke with a major seizure. Shortly

afterward, his physician arranged for a CAT scan of his brain; it revealed a large tumor located in an area where surgery could not be done. The patient received a course of brain irradiation and several months later a repeat of his CAT scan showed disappearance of the brain tumor. With great relief and some cautious optimism, both the patient's family and physician looked forward to a return of the patient to his normal level of functioning. However, over the following several months, the patient became more withdrawn, irritable, appeared to lose interest in his usual activities, and stopped going to work. Finally, under the assumption that he was simply unable to adjust to his medical misfortune, the patient was referred for psychiatric treatment of his depression. During the initial interview with the psychiatrist, the patient appeared withdrawn, had little spontaneity, and looked depressed. He would not respond to prompting from his wife to talk about his feelings. While he wife was describing her views of the situation, the patient would begin to gaze blankly out the window, a behavior the wife felt confirmed his inability to face his problem. It would have been quite understandable if this patient had been treated as a psychological casualty. Certainly, the appearance of a brain tumor in a middle-aged family man is a catastrophe that could account for any number of possible reactions, including depression and denial. However, a more thorough medical and neuropsychiatric evaluation revealed several additional problems. Of some significance was the fact that measurement of blood levels of anticonvulsant medication revealed that they were excessively high and probably accounted for some of the feelings of fatigue and lethargy that the patient experienced. In addition, careful assessment by a neuropsychologist of the patient's brain function revealed significant impairments that were probably secondary to the tumor, or to the radiation treatment, or both. Specifically, the patient demonstrated an exceedingly short attention span, inability sequentially to organize visual information in an efficient manner, and loss of some ability to think rapidly of the names of objects. When these deficits were finally appreciated, a new view of many of the patient's symptoms emerged. The patient's hesitance to return to work was not due to lack of motivation, but rather was the result of frustration with his inability to perform tasks that were formerly so straightforward for him. He gazed out the window not because of a lack of interest in solving his problems, but because his attention span was so brief that he could not follow a prolonged conversation. Recognition that the patient's symptoms were not caused by depression but were the consequence of some physical brain impairment had important implications for his management and rehabilitation. Specifically, both the patient and family stopped thinking of him as being a "bad person" or a "psychological invalid" and began to consider him as a person with some specific deficits who needed to develop alternative strategies to function. For example, the wife and family realized that "pushing" the patient to do more only served unduly to stress his limited capacities. Instead, it was more efficient to help the patient focus first on some limited goals. Trying to do less became an eventual means of accomplishing more. By a concrete problem-solving approach to limited aspects of his work, he was slowly able to return to his former job on a part-time basis within a few months. His positive feeling of these accomplishments contributed to improvement of his mood as well.

It has been very challenging to unravel the neurochemical functions of the human brain. Some understanding of this area is important for the clinician since an awareness of these medical aspects of depression will influence referral patterns, attribution of symptoms, and development of treatment plans.

Much of our current understanding of the biology of depression rests on observations made over 30 years ago that patients taking reserpine for the treatment of hypertension developed a constellation of symptoms that appeared identical to those of severely depressed psychiatric patients. Because reserpine was known to exert its antihypertensive effects by depleting a particular class of neurotransmitters known as catecholamines, it was hypothesized that depression also resulted from a lack of these neurotransmitters. Since that time, there has been a wealth of data in support of the notion that biogenic amine neurotransmitters play a significant role in vulnerability to and onset of major depression. Recently, possible biologic markers for depression have been reported. A significant portion of psychiatric patients with major depression have been found to have abnormalities in response to several tests of neuroendocrine function (notably the Dexamethasone Suppression Test) (Carroll et al. 1981) and the TRH stimulation test (Loosen and Prange 1982). Other indicators of biologic brain impairment in major depression include abnormalities in sleep physiology that can be documented using special sleep studies (McCarley 1982; Sitaram et al. 1982). Furthermore, it has become clear that the vulnerability to depression has a genetic basis

(Weitkamp et al. 1981). While the risk of developing a major depressive episode in the general population is somewhat less than 2%, it rises to approximately 16% in the first-degree relatives of those who have had major depression.

Despite the rapid progress in our understanding of the biology of depression, it is not yet possible to diagnose "major" depression in medical patients using a simple laboratory test in the way that other medical disorders are diagnosed. Yet the identification of a major depression is important as it implies that antidepressant medication should be considered as an adjunctive component of treatment. On what basis then does the validity of the diagnosis of depression rest? Basically, the clinician depends on the identification of a constellation of clinical signs and symptoms in the patient. There has been agreement recently upon a set of criteria for clinicians to follow in making the diagnosis of a major depressive episode. These have been published as part of a standardized diagnostic manual of the American Psychiatric Association, the DSM-III (1980). Clinicians should be aware that the DSM-III, as well as most of the psychometric instruments used in research on depression, were designed for use in psychiatric, nonmedically ill populations. Scores indicating the presence of depression from commonly used depression scales are all scaled in a way that somatic items can be a significant contribution to the overall score. To meet the criteria for the diagnosis of a major depressive episode, a medical patient should have a prominently and persistently depressed mood, not simple depressive feelings that occur from time to time and last only hours to a few days. In addition, there should be other features, including loss of interest or pleasure in usual activities; feelings of worthlessness, self-reproach, or excessive guilt; impaired concentration or thinking; suicidal ideation; or being speeded up or slowed down in thinking or movement. Symptoms such as sleep and appetite disturbance or fatigue are less useful in medically ill patients because they are often direct manifestations of the cancer or its treatment.

The Use of Antidepressants in Cancer Patients

There have been, to date, no published studies documenting the efficacy or special role of antidepressants in cancer patients specifically. In the absence of such research, there is as yet no way to predict what type of patients, with what symptoms, will respond to antidepressants. Nevertheless, it is generally appreciated on clinical grounds that antidepressants are effective in many depressed cancer patients. Many clinicians feel that when no medical cause can be found, depression represents a psychological process that should be addressed solely by psychotherapy or counseling, and not with medication. In fact, in some circles outright indignation may be expressed about the thought of using antidepressant medication in such circumstances since it is believed to imply that depressive symptoms are a "disease" rather than an understandable reaction to life circumstances. There also may be concern that "psychiatric" intervention might stigmatize the patient as having a psychiatric disorder rather than helping the person understand the meaning and context of the symptoms so as to resolve them. Depressed patients should be engaged in psychological treatments individually and with their families (DiMascio et al. 1979; Rush et al. 1982). However, antidepressants should be considered when symptoms remain unabated, especially if the symptoms include difficulty in sleeping, difficulty in concentrating, and feelings of being increasingly defeated and pessimistic. Some patients actually may prefer medication and object to a "nonmedical" psychological counseling approach since they may not be accustomed to thinking of themselves as candidates for psychological therapy. If patients are identified as having had a previous documented episode of depression, or if there is a strong family history of depression, there may be an even higher likelihood of potential benefit from an antidepressant medication. Once antidepressants are started, the first thing many patients begin to report is improvement in sleeping. When patients sleep better and feel more rested, they are usually able to think more clearly and feel more energetic. In addition, some patients report an increased sense of optimism and an improved sense of well-being. In the absence of a strict research design, it is, of course, impossible to know whether such improvements are attributable to a placebo effect, are secondary to being more rested, or are the result of any true mood-elevating effect of the antidepressant medication.

Despite the recognition that depression is a significant and prevalent problem for cancer patients, studies of the use of antidepressants in this population reveal that they account for only about 1% of the psychotropic drugs prescribed (Derogatis et al. 1979).

In general, oncologists are not familiar with using antidepressants and will tend to prescribe tranquilizing medication whenever a person seems distressed (Derogatis et al. 1979). Unfortunately, the use of tranquilizers such as diazepam (Valium) in depressed patients usually results only in a deeping of the depression, and possibly the unnecessary superimposition of some confusion.

General Principles of Clinical Use

Although the prescription and monitoring of antidepressants require a physician who is familiar with their use, some general understanding of treatment issues will be of use to the nonmedical clinician. Details concerning antidepressants are generally available (Hollister 1978a, b).

Despite some interesting scientific leads, there is no general agreement on a clinical or laboratory method to determine which antidepressant is best for a particular patient. If the patient had previously taken and responded to an antidepressant, there is a high likelihood of a repeat response to the same medication. If a first-degree relative has been successfully treated with an antidepressant, it is likely that the patient will respond in a similar fashion. If there is no such history, one is left with choosing a particular agent on the basis of its secondary features. For example, doxepin (Sinequan, Adapin) is said to have fewer cardiovascular effects but is somewhat more sedating than the others. Desipramine (Pertofrane, Norpramin) apparently has low anticholinergic potency and is among the least sedating, though some people find it makes them feel too "wired up." Deseryl (Trazadone) has virtually no anticholinergic activity. Protriptyline (Vivactil) may be used when excessive sedation is a special problem for the patient. As a general principle, it is important to use one medication for a long enough time at a high enough dose before drawing any conclusions about its effects. A common error, which is a great disservice to the patient, is to switch drugs before an adequate trial is given. Recent studies of antidepressant blood levels indicate a large range of plasma levels among different patients on the same oral dose (Hollister 1982). The implication is that while some patients may respond to as little as 25 or 50 mg. of an antidepressant, others require doses as high as 300 or 350 mg. Furthermore, there is evidence that, at least for nortriptyline (Aventyl), there is a "therapeutic window"; that is, lack of response may result from too high as well as too low a dose. Therefore, it is important to start at a low dose and gradually increase it. Starting at low doses also avoids unnecessary hypotension (which can lead to feelings of lightheadedness or dizziness) or oversedation.

While dose must be individualized, usually it is best to start treatment with 25 to 50 mg. at bedtime [except in the case of protriptyline, for which the dose is much lower than that of other tricyclics, and for deseryl (Trazadone), for which the dose is double that of other tricyclics]. After several days, the dose may be increased in increments of 25 to 50 mg. daily until a dose of about 150 mg. is reached. Because of their increased sensitivity to side effects, elderly patients, as well as those with CNS damage, should be treated with doses beginning in the range of 10 to 25 mg. per day. If a good clinical trial of one medication is not effective, it makes sense to change to another antidepressant that is least similar pharmacologically. Antidepressants do not work as aspirin does for a headache. When one has a headache, one expects aspirin to bring relief almost immediately. An antidepressant effect is usually not apparent until one to two weeks of treatment have passed. Too short a treatment period or too low a dose may be the cause of treatment failure. A single dose taken in the evening is generally as effective as divided doses, and may help the insomnia that is often prominent in depressed patients. These medications are not addicting.

Specifics of Antidepressant Medication

A number of drug types are available for the treatment of depression. These include tricyclic and tetracyclic antidepressants, the monoamine-oxidase (MAO) inhibitors, and the stimulants. Of these types of drugs, the tricyclic and tetracyclic antidepressants are by far the most commonly used, and probably the most effective. In general, there is no clear clinical indication for the use of stimulants (such as amphetamines), especially in light of their high abuse potential. However, as discussed in chapter 6, Pain, the addition of small amounts of stimulant medications such as amphetamine or methylphenidate (Ritalin) can be exceedingly beneficial as they appear to augment analgesia (Forrest et al. 1977) as well as to provide some mood-elevating properties. In older patients who are depressed and anergic, small doses of stimulant medication in the morning are considered by some a viable depression treatment approach. At this time, however, it seems that relatively little is known about this practice. Because the MAO inhibitors are associated with a myriad of dangerous drug interactions and side effects, their use is somewhat restricted and should not be considered a first-line treatment in this population. The properties of tricyclic antidepressants were first noted in 1957 and the first member, imipramine (Tofranil), was marketed in 1958. The continued search for related compounds has led to a large number of additional antidepressants and other chemical families now available and in wide use. Over the next few years, the patient may benefit from "second generation" antidepressants, which are as effective as the tricyclics and appear to have fewer side effects. The antidepressants that are most widely used at the present time include those shown in Table 4.2.

Antidepressant Drug Interactions and Side Effects

Sedative Effects

The sedative effects of antidepressants are among their most common and bothersome side effects. Such sedative effects are additive with all other sedatives, including alcohol and the sedating effects of narcotic analgesics. However, oversedation usually can be avoided by custom tailoring the dose to the individual or by switching to another, less sedating agent. The sedative properties of antidepressants, which are most marked soon after taking a single dose, can be taken advantage of as a remedy for insomnia. For this reason, antidepressants are often best taken in a single daily dose just before bedtime. The sedation often wears off by the morning, while the antidepressant effects themselves continue on through the day. Elderly patients seem especially sensitive to this effect and may easily become oversedated and confused on surprisingly small doses of tricyclics. Certainly, no cancer patient needs this additional burden. For this reason, some physicians are inclined to consider the relative sedative properties of antidepressants in their prescribing (see Table 4.2).

TABLE 4.2
Identification of Antidepressants

ANTIDEPRESSANT	RELATIVE ANTICHOLINERGIC POTENCY	RELATIVE SEDATIVE ACTIVITY
Tricyclic Tertiary Amines		
Amitriptyline (Elavil; Endep)	⫴⫼	⫴⫼
Imipramine (Tofranil)	⫴⫼	⫴⫼
Doxepin (Sinequan, Adapin)	⫴⫼	⫴⫼⫴
Trimipramine (Surmontil)	⫴⫼	⫴⫼
Tricyclic Secondary Amines		
Desimipramine (Norpramin, Pertofrane)	+	+
Nortriptyline (Aventyl)	⫴⫼	⫴⫼
Protriptyline (Vivactil)	⫴⫼⫴	+
Tetracyclics		
Maprotiline (Ludiomil)	+	⫴⫼
Tricyclic Dibenzoxazepines		
Amoxapine (Asendin)	+	⫴⫼
Triazolopyridines		
Trazadone (Deseryl)	0	⫴⫼

Anticholinergic Effects

Tricyclic and tetracyclic antidepressants interfere with acetylcholine, which is one of the major neurotransmitters in both the central and peripheral nervous system. These resulting effects account for many of the common adverse problems associated with the use of these agents. Dry mouth is the most common side effect and seems to be unavoidable, though it is usually more of a nuisance than a danger to patients. The simplest way to deal with this is to have the patient suck on some sugarless mints. Constipation is another common side effect of this medication, thus adding to the constipation problems of those on narcotics for pain. Because of anticholinergic effects, these drugs should not be used in patients with narrow-angle glaucoma or prostatic hypertrophy (since urinary retention can be precipitated). Patients who have spinal cord involvement are especially prone to this group of side effects that can lead to disruption of bladder function and loss of bowel function. At excessive doses, anticholinergic effects can lead to increased confusion and delirium. The appearance of increasing confusion in any patient on antidepressants should lead to their temporary discontinuation. Anticholinergic effects are additive with drugs having similar effects. States of confusion are often precipitated by combinations of tricyclics with such drugs as atropine, used in eye drops or anesthesia, meperidine (Demerol), and antispasmodics such as Donnatal and propantheline (Pro-Banthine) used for gastrointestinal disorders.

Cardiovascular Effects

The effects of antidepressants on the heart are the most controversial and potentially dangerous consequences (Bigger et al 1978). Because of changes in conduction of electrical impulses within the heart and alteration of extrinsic nervous regulation of heart rate, there is potential for a wide variety of problems in heart rate, rhythm, and overall function. Certainly any cancer patient beginning on an antidepressant should have an electrocardiogram to screen for conduction disorders that would rule out the use of antidepressants. Tricyclics should not be used for several months following a myocardial infarction. People who already have some impairment in cardiac condition are at risk for either further block or precipitation of an arrhythmia. People with certain arrhythmias are actually improved by the effects of antidepressants, since some of them act like quinidine, a drug used to decrease the tendency to develop abnormal rhythms (Bigger et al. 1977). These factors must all be carefully considered, though many cardiac conditions do not preclude the use of antidepressants (Veith et al. 1982).

Orthostatic hypotension is another common cardiovascular effect. This results in a feeling of lightheadedness and dizziness when getting up from a lying or sitting position. Such posture-induced changes in blood pressure may be quite serious and lead to injuries from falling. Finally, patients should be aware that antidepressants can block the effect of antihypertensives such as guanethidine (Ismelin), methyldopa (Aldomet), and clonidine (Catapres).

Psychiatric Consultation

A psychiatric consultant can often play an important role in the assessment of a disturbed or disturbing cancer patient by making the diagnosis, whether it be an underlying organic mental disorder or depression, assisting in its differential evaluation (including its separation from other psychiatric syndromes or adjustment reactions), and planning treatment. Unfortunately, medical patients, their families, and some professional providers often attach an unnecessary stigma to psychiatric consultation. Failure to recognize and treat an organic mental disorder or major depression can result in unnecessary alienation of the patient from friends and environment as well as premature loss of functional status. A psychiatric referral is often misperceived as implying that the patient's difficulties are "all in the head" or that the patient is a "mental case." On the contrary, psychiatric consultation provides an important dimension to medical care inasmuch as the psychiatrist is trained to evaluate and diagnose those biomedical disorders that can mimic psychological or psychosocial disturbances.

Diagnostic medical studies commonly employed in the search for specific etiologies of OMD may include blood tests, a spinal tap, EEG, and CAT scans. Primary treatment consists of identification and correction of the underlying medical abnormality. In addition, certain adjunctive treatment measures are often helpful. Small doses of neuroleptic medication (such as haloperidol) may be helpful in controlling the agitation of a confused patient. Environmental manipulations are often overlooked despite their significant impact on minimizing patient confusion. Confused patients often can improve remarkably when provided with orienting cues such as large, readable calendars and clocks, along with night lights, familiar objects from home, and frequent verbal orientation by staff and family. Clear, straightforward, and consistent communication from the staff and family will also help the patients organize their experience. It should never be assumed that confused patients cannot participate in their treatment. Instead, the counselor should encourage physicians and family to help engage the patient by repetition, clarity, and a *slower pace* of communication. Confused patients must be carefully prepared for changes in treatment, procedures, or location rather than treated as though they do not know what is happening. Delirium can represent a frightening and stressful life event for the patient. Therefore, after its resolution, it may be useful to discuss what happened with the patient, providing assurance that the patient did not lose his mind or have an emotional illness. (Mackenzie and Popkin 1980).

Because so many of the symptoms involved with depression can be produced directly as the result of medical illness or its treatment, the diagnosis of depression in medical patients becomes problematic and may require psychiatric consultation. Naturally there are a large variety of psychological and psychosocial issues that often sufficiently explain why such a person appears depressed. These issues are discussed at length in other chapters. Psychological adjustment issues are always an important part of the management of patients with severe medical illness, whether or not other biologic components can be identified and addressed. However, the most frequent error in the evaluation of such symptoms is to assume that the psychological explanation is sufficient. "Wouldn't you be depressed if you had cancer?" is often used as a disclaimer for further evaluation. Depression must be regarded as a nonspecific symptom that requires careful systematic evaluation in the same way as nonspecific medical symptoms such as anemia, jaundice, and fever.

All patients with significant symptoms of depression should be carefully evaluated for the possibility of underlying medical conditions that can produce the symptoms. If any of these factors can be identified, correction of the underlying medical condition must be undertaken. In many cases, the symptoms of depression will resolve. In others, one must decide whether or not to supplement a psychosocial treatment approach with the use of antidepressant medication. Virtually every study of depression in cancer patients has been hampered by the limitations of applying psychiatric diagnostic criteria to a medical population. Several findings, however, are consistently clear. Careful review of cancer patients labeled as having depression have consistently shown a high incidence of misdiagnoses with oversight of underlying organic medical problems. It also appears that empiric use of tricyclic antidepressants, if not medically contraindicated, can be a helpful adjunct in the treatment of depression. Naturally, psychotropic medications cannot change underlying personality problems or the harsh realities of misfortune that may precipitate psychosocial adjustment problems; however, they often can alleviate symptoms that impair the person's innate coping resources and allow a more effective grappling with adverse circumstances.

References

ALLEN, J. C.: The effects of cancer therapy on the nervous system. *J. Pediatr.* 93 (1978): 903–909.

American Psychiatric Association: *Diagnostic and statistical manual of mental disorders* (third edition), 1980.

ANDERSON, A. E., AND McHUGH, P. R.: Oat cell carcinoma with hypercortisolemia presenting to a psychiatric hospital as a suicide attempt. *J. Nerv. Ment. Dis.* 152 (1971): 427–431.

ARMSTRONG, D., YOUNG, L. S., MEYER, R. D., ET AL. Infectious complications of neoplastic disease. *Med. Clin. N. Am.* 55 (1971): 729–745.

BARRON, K. D., SIGUEIRA, E., AND HIRANO, A.: Cerebral embolism caused by nonbacterial thrombotic endocarditis. *Neurology* 10 (1976): 391–397.

BIGGER, J., KANTOR, S. J., GLASSMAN, A. H., AND PEREL, J. M.: Cardiovascular effects of tricyclic antidepressant drugs. In M. A. Lipton, A. DiMascio, and K. F. Killam (Eds.), *Psychopharmacology: A generation of progress*. New York: Raven Press, 1978.

BIGGER, J. T., JR., GIARDINA, E. G. V., PEREL, J. M. ET AL.: Cardiac antiarrhythmic effects of imipramine hydrochloride. *N. Engl. J. Med.* 296 (1977): 206–208.

BLEYER, W. A.: Methotrexate: Clinical pharmacology current status and therapeutic guidelines. *Cancer Treat Rev.* 4 (1977): 87.

BRYAN, C. S.: Nonbacterial thrombotic endocarditis with malignant tumors. *Am. J. Med.* (1969): 787–793.

CARROLL, B. F., FEINBERG, M., GREDEN, J. F., TARIKA, J., ALBALA, A. A.; HASKETT, R. F., JAMES, N. M., KRONFOL, Z., LOHR, N., STEINER, M., DE VIGNE, J. P., AND YOUNG, E.: A specific laboratory test for the diagnosis of melancholia. *Arch. Ger. Psychiatry* 38 (1981): 15–22.

CARROLL, B. J.: Psychiatric disorders and steroids. In E. Usdin, D. A. Hamburg, and J. D. Barchas (Eds.), *Neuroregulators and psychiatric disorders*. Oxford: Oxford University Press, 1977, chap. 31.

CHERNIK, N. L., ARMSTRONG, D., AND POSNER, J. B.: Central nervous system infections in patients with cancer. *Medicine* 52 (1978): 563–580.

CRAIG, T. J., AND ABELOFF, M. D.: Psychiatric symptomatology among hospitalized cancer patients. *Am. J. Psychiatry* 131 (1974): 1323–1327.

CORSELLIS, J. A. N.: Subacute encephalitis and malignancy. In C. W. M. Whitty, J. T. Hughes, and F. O. MacCallum (Eds.), *Vi-*

rus diseases of the nervous system. Oxford: Blackwell Scientific Publications, 1969, pp. 207–212.

CROFT, P. B., AND WILKINSON, M.: The incidence of carcinomatous neuromyopathy with special reference to carcinoma of the lung and breast. In W. R. Brain, and F. H. Norris (Eds.), *The remote effects of cancer on the nervous system.* New York: Grune & Stratton, 1965.

DEROGATIS, L. R., FELDSTEIN, M., MORROW, G. ET AL.: A survey of psychotropic drug prescriptions in an oncology population. *Cancer* 44 (1979): 1919–1929.

DEROGATIS, L. R., MORROW G. R., FETTING J., ET AL.: The Prevalence of Psychiatric Disorders Among Cancer Patients. *JAMA* 249 (1983): 751–757.

DIMASCIO, A., WEISSMAN, M. M., PRUSOFF, B. A., NEU, C., ZWILLING, M., AND KLERMAN, G. L.: Differential symptom reduction by drugs and psychotherapy in acute depression. *Arch. Gen. Psychiatry* 36 (1979): 1450–1456.

ENGEL, G. L., AND ROMANO, J.: Delirium, a syndrome of cerebral insufficiency. *J. Chron. Dis.* 9 (1959): 260–276.

EPSTEIN, B. S., EPSTEIN, J. A., AND POSTEL, D. M.: Tumors of spinal cord simulating psychiatric disorders. *Dis. Nerv. Syst.* 32 (1971): 741–743.

FOLSTEIN, M., AND MCHUGH, P.: "Mini-mental state." A practical method for grading the cognitive state of patients for the clinician. *J. Psychiatr. Res.* 12 (1975): 189–198.

FORREST, W. H. ET AL.: Dextroamphetamine with morphine for the treatment of postoperative pain. *N. Engl. J. Med.* 296 (1977): 712.

GEHI, M. H., ROSENTHAL, R. H., FIZETTE, N. B., ET AL.: Psychiatric manifestions of hyponatremia. *Psychosomatics* 22 (1981): 739–743.

GOLDBERG, I. D., BLOOMER, W. D., DAWSON, D. M.: Nervous system toxic effects of cancer therapy. *JAMA* 247 (1982): 1437–1441.

GOLDBERG, R. J.: *Anxiety: A guide to biobehavioral diagnosis and therapy for physicians and mental health clinicians.* Garden City, N.Y.: Medical Examination Publishing Co., 1982.

————: Management of depression in the patient with advanced cancer. *JAMA* 246 (July 24, 31, 1981): 373–376.

HALL, R. C. W., AND JOFFE, J. R.: Hypomagnesemia: Physical andpsychiatric symptoms. *JAMA* 224 (1973): 1749–1751.

HALL, R. C. W., POPKIN, M. K., DEVAUL, R. A., ET AL.: Physical illness presenting as psychiatric disease. *Arch. Gen. Psychiatry* 35 (1978): 1315–1320.

HECAEN, H., AND AJURIAGUERRA, S. DE: *Troubles mentaux du cours des tumours intracraniennes.* Paris: Masson, 1956.

HINTON, J.: The psychiatry of terminal illness in adults and children. *Proc. Roy. Soc. Med.* 65 (1972): 1035–1040.

HOCHBERG, F.: Neurological aspects of systemic tumors. In K. J. Isselbacher, and R. D. Adams (Eds.), *Principles of internal medicine* (9th edi.). Update I, New York: McGraw-Hill, 1981.

HOFFMAN, R. S.: Diagnostic Errors in the Evaluation of Behavioral Disorders. *JAMA* 248 (1982): 964–967.

HOLLISTER, L. E.: Plasma concentrations of tricyclic antidepressants in clinical practice. *J. Clin. Psychiatry* 43 (1982): 66–69.

———: Tricyclic antidepressants (first of two parts). *N. Engl. J. Med.* 299 (1978): 1106–1110.

———: Tricyclic antidepressants (second of two parts). *N. Engl. J. Med.* 299 (1978): 1168–1172.

KESCHNER, M., BENDER, M. B., AND STRAUSS, I.: Mental symptoms in cases of tumor of the temporal lobe. *Arch. Neurol. Psychiatry* 35 (1936): 572–596.

KLATCHKO, B., GORZYNSKI, J. G., BURTEN, W., ET AL.: A Prospective controlled study of depression. In Patients with pancreatic cancer and other intrabdominal malignancies. *Psychosomatic Med.* 44 (July 1982): 301, abstract.

KNIGHTS, E. B., AND FOLSTEIN, M. S.: Unsuspected emotional and cognitive disturbance in medical patients. *Ann. Intern. Med.* 87 (1977): 723–724.

KORANYI, E. K.: Morbidity and rate of undiagnosed physical illnesses in a psychiatric clinic population. *Arch. Gen. Psychiatry* 36 (1979): 414–419.

LEVINE, P. M., SILBERFARB, P. M., AND LIPOWSKI, Z. J.: Mental disorders in cancer patients. A study of 100 psychiatric referrals. *Cancer* 42 (1978): 1385–1391.

LING, M. H. M., PERRY, P. J., AND TSUANG, M. T.: Side effects of corticosteroid therapy. *Arch. Gen. Psychiatry* 38 (1981): 471–477.

LOOSEN, P. T., AND PRANGE, A. J.: Serum thyrotropin response to thyrotropin-releasing hormone in psychiatric patients: A review. *Am. J. Psychiatry* 139 (1982): 405–416.

MCCARLEY, R. W.: REM sleep and depression: Common neurobiological control mechanisms. *Am. J. Psychiatry* 139 (1982): 565–570.

MACKENZIE, T. B., POPKIN, M. K.: Psychological manifestations of nonbacterial thrombotic endocarditis. *Am. J. Psychiatry* 137 (1980): 1433–1435.

MALAMUD, N.: Psychiatric disorder with intracranial tumors of thelimbic system. *Arch. Neurol.* 17 (1967): 113–128.

MEADOWS, A. T., MASSARI, D. J., FERGUSSON, J., ET AL.: Declines in IQ scores and cognitive dysfunctions in children with acute lymphocytic leukaemia treated with cranial irradiation. *Lancet* II (1981): 1015-1018.

MITCHINSON, M. J.: The hypotensive stroke. *Lancet* (1980): 244-246.

Moss, H. A., NANNIS, E. D., AND POPLACK, D. G.: The effects of prophylactic treatment of the central nervous system on the intellectual functioning of children with acute lymphocytic leukemia. *Am. J. Med.* 71 (1981): 47-52.

PECK, A.: Emotional reactions to having cancer. *J. Roentgenol. Radium Ther. Nucl. Med.* 114 (1972): 591-599.

PLUMB, M. M., AND HOLLAND, J.: Comparative studies of psychological factors in patients with advanced cancer. *J. Psychosom. Med.* 39 (1977): 264-276.

POSNER, J. B.: Neurological complications of systemic cancer. *Med. Clin. N. Am.* 55: 625-646, 1971.

PULLAN, P. T., CLEMENT-JONES, V., CORDER, R., ET AL.: Ectopic production of methionine enkephalin and beta-endorphin. *Br. Med. J.* I (1980): 758-759.

RALSTON, S., GARDNER, M. D., FOGELMAN, I., ET AL.: Hypercalcaemia and metastatic bone disease: Is there a causal link? *Lancet* Oct. 23, 1982: 903-905.

REAGAN, T. J., OKAZAKI, H.: The thrombotic syndrome associated with carcinoma. *Arch. Neurol.* 31: 390-395, 1974.

ROSEN, P. R., AND ARMSTRONG, D.: Nonbacterial thrombotic endocarditis in patients with malignant neoplastic diseases. *Am. J. Med.* 54: 23-29, 1973.

RUSH, A. J., BECK, A. T., KOVACS, M., WEISSENBURGER, J., AND HOLLON, S. D.: Comparison of the effects of cognitive therapy and pharmacotherapy on hopelessness and self-concept. *Am. J. Psychiatry* 139 (1982): 862-866.

SCHAFER, D. F., AND JONES, E. A.: Hepatic encephalopathy and the y-aminobutyric-acid neurotransmitter system. *Lancet* (1982): 18-20.

SEGALOFF, A.: Managing endocrine and metabolic problems in the patient with advanced cancer. *JAMA* 245 (1981): 177-179.

SHAPIRO, W. R.: Remote effects of neoplasm on central nervous system: Encephalopathy. In R. A. Thompson, and J. R. Green (Eds.), *Advances in neurology*, volume 15. New York: Raven Press, 1976.

SHELINE, G. E.: Irradiation Injury of the Human Brain: A Review of Clinical Experience. Chapter in H. A. Gilbert, and A. R. Kagan

(Eds.), *Radiation Damage to the Nervous System*. New York: Raven Press, 1980.

SHERWOOD, L. M.: The multiple causes of hypercalcemia in malignant disease. *N. Engl. J. Med.* 303 (1980): 1412–1413.

SITARAM, N., NURNBERGER, J. I., GERSHON, E. S., AND GILLIN, J. C.: Cholinergic regulation of mood and REM sleep: Potential model and marker of vulnerability of affective disorder. *Am. J. Psychiatry* 139 (1982): 571–576.

STEWART, A. F., HORST, R., DEFTOS, L. J., ET AL.: Biochemical evaluation of patients with cancer-associated hypercalcemia. *N. Engl. J. Med* 303 (1980): 1377–1383.

STRAUSS, I., AND KESCHNER, M.: Mental symptoms in cases of tumor of the frontal lobe. *Arch. Neurol. Psychiatry* 33 (1935): 986–1005.

THORSON, A., HANSON, A., PERNOW, B., ET AL.: Carcinoid tumor within an ovarian teratoma in a patient with a carcinoid syndrome (carcinoidosis). *Acta Med. Scand.* 161 (suppl. 334 1958): 495–505.

VEITH, R. C., RASKIND, M. A., CALDWELL, J. H., ET AL.: Cardiovascular effects of tricyclic antidepressants in depressed patients with chronic heart disease. *N. Engl. J. Med.* 306 (1982): 954–959.

WEBB, W. L., AND GEHI, M.: Electrolyte and fluid imbalance: Neuropsychiatric manifestations. *Psychosomatics* 22 (1981): 199–203.

WEIL, A. A.: Ictal emotions occurring in temporal lobe dysfunction. *Arch. Neurol.* 1: 87–97, 1959.

WEITKAMP, L. R., STANCER, H. C., PERSAD, E., FLOOD, C., AND GUTTORMSEN, S.: Depressive disorders and HLA: A gene on chromosome 6 that can affect behavior. *N. Engl. J. Med.* 305 (1981): 1301–1306.

WEIZMAN, A., ELDAR, M. SCHOENFELD, Y., ET AL.: Hypercalcemia-induced psychopathology in malignant diseases. *Br. J. Psychiatry* 135 (1979): 363–366.

WILLIAMS, M., AND PENNYBACKER, J. B.: Memory disturbances in third ventricle tumors. *J. Neurol. Neurosurg. Psychiatry* 17 (1954): 115–123.

WONG, E. T., AND FREIER, E. F.: The Differential diagnosis of hypercalcemia: An algorithm for more effective use of laboratory tests. *JAMA* 247 (1982): 75–80.

YAHR, M. D., DUVOISIN, R. C., AND COWEN, D.: Encephalopathy associated with carcinoma. *Trans. Am. Neurol. Assoc.* 90 (1965): 80–86.

CHAPTER 5

Psychiatric Aspects of Medication

PATIENTS WITH SIGNIFICANT medical illness are regularly exposed to a large number of medications with potential psychiatric consequences (Davidson et al. 1975; Salzman 1981). (See Table 5.1.) In the medical setting, the unrecognized effects of drugs probably account for a significant number of problems that are mistakenly considered to be psychological in nature. Reviews of the prescribing practices of physicians treating cancer patients show that the majority of their patients are usually on more than one medication that affects the central nervous system (CNS) (Derogatis et al. 1979). In fact, the three drugs most commonly prescribed in the United States today, cimetidine (Tagament), propranolol (Inderal), and diazepam (Valium) are all known to produce a variety of disorders of mood, thought, and behavior including psychosis, confusion, depression, and irritability. As the number of medications increases, drug interactions rise geometrically, thus creating an increased likelihood of an adverse psychiatric effect. As a general principle, patients should be on the lowest dose of the fewest medications for the shortest possible time.

111

TABLE 5.1
Drugs Reported to Produce Psychiatric Symptoms

Analgesics	*Chemotherapeutic Agents*
Indomethacin (Indocin)	5-Fluorouracil
Meperidine (Demerol)	L-asparaginase
Pentazocine (Talwin)	Mechlorethamine
Propoxyphene (Darvon)	Methotrexate
	Steroids
Anesthetics	Vinblastine
Ketamine	Vincristine
Lidocaine	
Phencyclidine (PCP)	*CNS Sedatives*
	All (associated with intoxication
	or withdrawal), especially
Anticholinergic Agents	alcohol, barbiturates,
Antidepressants	benzodiazepines
Antihistamines	
Anti-Parkinson agents	
e.g. Benztropine (Cogentin)	*CNS Stimulants*
Antispasmodics	Amphetamine
e.g. propantheline	Cocaine
(Pro-Banthine)	Ephedrine
Atropine	Methylphenidate (Ritalin)
Phenothiazines	
	Dopaminergic Drugs
Anticonvulsants	Amantadine (Symmetrel)
All (at high doses)	Bromocriptine
	Levodopa (L-Dopa)
Antihypertensives	
Methyldopa (Aldomet)	*Miscellaneous*
Prazosin (Minipress)	Amphotericin-B
Propranolol (Inderal)	Baclofen
Reserpine	Cimetidine (Tagamet)
Thiazide diuretics	Digitalis

Common, though avoidable, psychiatric side effects of medication arise from four factors: (1) a general lack of awareness of the behavioral consequences of many commonly used drugs; (2) a tendency to overprescribe; (3) failure to discontinue drugs when they are no longer indicated; and (4) a lack of understanding of the pharmacologic properties of many medications. Both the patient and physician share some responsibility for this state of affairs since the overuse of drugs is at times due to unrealistic patient expectations that there is a "pill" for everything. As it is a virtual certainty that medical patients at some time will be given a medication that affects the CNS, this chapter presents an overview of some of the typical problems that will be encountered. Recognition that symptoms such as confusion, anxiety, depression, lethargy, or agitation may in fact be drug side effects has crucial importance for the patient and family since proper recognition avoids unnecessary suffering and functional impairment.

The Experience of Taking Many Medications

With society's increasing emphasis on health and natural values, the sudden confrontation with an illness that necessitates taking not one but many medications can be very disturbing. General feelings and attitudes toward medication are starkly challenged when the patient is confronted with the recommendation to begin chemotherapy—a treatment which, for many people, has a reputation for being a cure worse than the disease. Public reservations about chemotherapy have certainly been reinforced by current media attention that may lead some to infer that patients are dying from the treatment and not the cancer. Certainly the person who says "I never took anything in my life, and think that pill users are poisoning themselves" is in for a problem when faced with catastrophic illness. It is important for the physician to be aware of such attitudes and patterns of medication behavior since they will surely influence the treatment process. It is unfortunate that people sometimes find themselves caught up in an empty conflict between being "prodrug" and "antidrug" when the appropriate use of drugs is the issue. Anxiety about the illness sometimes becomes displaced and focused around an exaggerated concern about taking medication. When a patient complains of having to, but not liking to, take medications, clinicians should be careful to examine their own feelings about medication before responding. What the clinicians might feel about a medication or do for themselves is not always appropriate for the patient. For those clinicians who are somewhat antimedication, it is important to elicit the patient's specific concerns about medication rather than automatically to commiserate or support a negative attitude.

The use of medication is a complex process with psychological and interpersonal elements. The high rates of noncompliance with prescriptions is well known. For example, it has been estimated that between 25 and 50% of the time there is complete failure to take any of the prescriptions written for outpatients (Blackwell 1972). What accounts for this incredible gap between the pen and the lip? Secret fears, beliefs based on hearsay, misinterpretation of some confusing experience, family and social attitudes, as well as feelings about the physician, all play major roles (Byck 1978). Because it has been recognized that accurate factual information improves patient compliance, many programs have begun to devote some resources to patient education by making printed literature available or having a pharmacist meet with the patient. However, despite the importance of accurate information, an educational approach remains naive about the more powerful subterranean factors that determine drug-taking behaviors. The availability of clear information is an important though insufficient step toward helping many patients whose ambivalence is based on private concerns not generally discussed. For example, if it is suggested that the patient take a steroid, she may say "That drug! A woman in my bridge group took that and she said that it made her arms hairy," or "A girl down the street from me was put on that just before she tried to kill herself and went to a mental hospital." Such responses are somewhat extreme but typify concerns over unknown adverse effects and giving up control to medication. If such feelings are not expressed and addressed in some way, the likelihood of taking enough medication to get a beneficial effect is markedly reduced. Other more conventional concerns are: "Will I become addicted?" "Will I become impotent?" "Will this put me to sleep during the day?" Getting the patient to take some initiative in communicating with the physician is an important part of taking medication. Giving the prescription to the patient is too often seen by the physician as the end of the process when it is clearly only the beginning of the experience for the patient. Taking medication is more like having a custom fitting for a suit than buying furniture. The eventual correct fit depends on sequential alterations determined by the unique physical characteristics of the patient, his or her sense of what looks and feels right, and the skills of the tailor in producing a finished product. The role of the nonmedical clinician in dealing with patients who have a problem with medication is to assist patients (and/or the patient's family) to become more active and effective in working with their physicians. Patients who are assisted out of a passive role are able to maintain some sense of control and participation in the medication process.

There may be people who feel they do not want to know anything about their medication, the reasons for it, or what it might do. In light of today's consumer-oriented culture, such an attitude might be viewed as regressive; however, little is actually known about the success of treatment experiences for such patients as compared with those who actively seek detailed information, or whether information can be harmful (Loftus and Fries 1979). It can be extremely frustrating to work with patients who make it clear that they do not want to know about the details of their treatment. On the surface, it would seem that the more passive the patient, the easier the clinical task. However, this is not so. The very passivity creates problems; some of these can be explained rationally, whereas others cannot. Patients who do not want to know about their treatment foster splitting in the care system since some people around them, such as family members, may want to know more. This discrepancy in information creates tension, secrets, and unnecessary problems that have to be dealt with. The excessively passive patient also may seem more like a victim. Such people, it is felt, may be more likely to die, since many clinicians have the attitude that it is crucial to have a "will to live." Such passivity is also unacceptable to action-oriented helpers who may become resentful that they are trying while the patient is not. Some clinicians feel that denial is inherently negative, yet may harbor their own wish at some level to be "kept in the dark," thus creating conflict in working with the patient. When the patient indicates or says directly to the treatment system, "Do what you want, but don't tell me about it," there is little use in meeting the problem head on and asking, "Why don't you want to hear more?" or "What are you afraid of?" If the patient were clearly in touch with the answers to such questions, he/she would be in a different situation to begin with. Instead, engaging the patient indirectly around problems that may be of concern (for example, by using parts of the semistructured interview from Appendix A) is a more useful approach that might hit on an underlying issue, or at least give the patient a positive experience of interacting with the helping professional, which may provide a foundation for future work together. Different levels of involvement seem appropriate for different personalities. Unfortunately, not every patient is going to find a physician who will be sensitive to these issues or take the initiative in such topics. However, many will be quite reasonable when concerns are brought to their attention in a reasonable way. If there is an extreme mismatch between the patient's needs for attention and physician's inclination to get involved in this area, the outcome of prescribing will certainly be less than optimal.

Once the Prescription Is Written . . .

Patients must be encouraged to take responsibility for reporting any adverse effects. It is unrealistic to expect the physician to anticipate the unique responses of every patient to every drug. The physician does have the responsibility to tell the patient about the most common adverse effects and the significant risks and benefits involved with a particular drug. However, everyone's body chemistry is unique in regard to a host of factors, including rate of metabolism, presence of other potentially interacting substances, and vulnerability to experience symptoms that influence behavior. But many patients (1) are afraid to bother the physician with "minor" problems such as side effects, (2) think adverse effects are unavoidable and must be put up with, (3) are made to feel that they should not call, or (4) are unaware of the relationships between certain adverse experiences and the medications they are taking. Such attitudes lead either to unnecessary suffering or to premature discontinuation of treatment. What should a nonmedical clinician working with the patient do upon observing that an important side effect maybe occurring and that neither the patient nor the physician seems aware of the problem? Calling the physician directly has its drawbacks as physicians frequently deal with visiting nurses or social workers abruptly, especially if the communication seems tentative—which it may be if the helping clinician feels unsure about what is going on medically. Further, calling the physician directly creates a split in the doctor–patient system and provides a negative model for the patient, who is made to feel powerless and ineffectual. Instead, the issue should be brought up with the patient (and/or family), who should than take the responsibility to deal with the physician. A nonmedical clinician can do extremely important work by assisting patients and families to resolve such problems with their physicians.

A related problem emerges when the patient becomes a student of the *PDR*. A widely used sourcebook of drug information, the *Physician's Desk Reference* (*PDR*) is a compendium of information inserts prepared by the marketing drug companies to comply with a variety of federal regulations. Unfortunately, the nature of the regulations requires listing of virtually every possible related side effect ever reported, making the *PDR* a poor (though accessible) reference source. Without some sense of perspective, the consumer is often overwhelmed and frightened by the panoply of devastating effects reported for almost every substance. While the motivation is correct, the outcome may be unexpectedly aversive.

It may be helpful for the nonphysician to have some idea of the physician's perspective. How much information should be shared with a patient about adverse effects? Telling a patient too little can be infantilizing, may deprive the patient of a sense of participation and choice, and is risky in a medicolegal sense. The patient's need for involvement in treatment is crucial, and lack of such a feeling may be one of the important factors that lead patients to seek unorthodox therapies (Cassileth 1982). If one assails the patient with the laundry list of potential catastrophes mentioned in the *PDR*, the fear is that the patient either will be frightened away (and thereby miss the opportunity for a cure) or will be so influenced by the power of suggestion that increased side effects may develop. But although a patient may be more uncomfortable following disclosure of possible side effects, such an outcome is considered unavoidable given current attitudes toward disclosure and informed consent. The physician often feels somewhat isolated and left on his/her own to make decisions about where to draw the line in introducing important information without creating excessive iatrogenic fears and preoccupations.

The Psychiatric Consequences of Medication

Recent reviews have compiled the large number of medications (see Table 5.1) associated with psychiatric consequences [also see Abromowicz (1981)].

Analgesics

Occasionally, idiosyncratic reactions seem to occur with narcotics, with symptoms which can include agitated behavior, delirium or hallucinations. It is often difficult to determine whether such symptoms are directly due to the narcotic or whether they are secondary to the concomitant factors of pain, sleep deprivation, and other medical stresses. Meperidine (Demerol), given in high doses, especially if there is renal impairment, can lead to symptoms of agitation and even seizures. Dysphoric reactions, including symptoms of depersonalization are not uncommon with combined narcotic agonists/antagonists such as pentazocine (Talwin), and for this reason this drug is best avoided. Extreme anxiety and agitation accompanies narcotic withdrawal and may be iatrogenically introduced by abrupt changes in narcotic orders. Chapter 6 contains a more detailed review of the analgesics.

Anticholinergics

Anticholinergic effects are shared by a wide variety of commonly used medications such as antihistamines and antidepressants. These effects cause changes in neurotransmission in the brain (as well as peripherally), which can lead to a syndrome consisting of confusion, memory loss, disorientation, depersonalization, delirium, auditory and visual hallucinations, fear, and paranoia as its psychiatric manifestations (Hall et al. 1981; Johnson et al. 1981). Single agents with enough anticholinergic activity can produce such symptoms when they accumulate, and patients on more than one drug with anticholinergic effects are at increased risk.

Anticonvulsants

Patients on anticonvulsants such as phenytoin (Dilantin) or phenobarbital can have a variety of psychiatric side effects if the levels are not monitored and maintained within the therapeutic range (Rivinus, 1982). Excessively high doses of phenytoin (Dilantin) actually can lead to hallucinations, delirium, agitation, depression, or confusion (Franks and Richter 1979; Tollefson 1980). It is not uncommon to see patients requiring several anticonvulsants to control the seizures associated with brain tumors or the sequelae of surgery for brain tumors. High levels of sedative anticonvulsants, such as the barbiturates or diazepam (Valium), can make the patient feel increasingly depressed and lethargic. At times, it is difficult to sort this out from a psychological reaction to the disease itself. Whenever this is in question, one should arrange for plasma levels to be obtained to make sure the patient is within the therapeutic range.

Antihypertensives

Including methyldopa (Aldomet), reserpine, propranolol (Inderal), and prazosin (Minipress), have been associated with effects on brain neurotransmitters that lead to clinically significant depression as well as fatigue, confusion, and impotence (Paykel et al. 1982). When a patient on one of these medications becomes depressed, it is difficult to state that it is "due to" the antihypertensives. However, in most cases, it is useful to arrange for the patient to change medications to one not associated with depression. Patients on diuretics such as furosemide (Lasix) or thiazides should have their potassium levels checked periodically as low potassium can lead to weakness, decreased motivation, and confusion, as well as some serious medical consequences.

Stimulants

Caffeine is one of the most widely used psychotropic drugs in the United States. In a survey of caffeine use, approximately 25% of respondents reported using greater than 500 to 600 mg of caffeine per day (Abelson and Fishburne 1976). The approximate amount of caffeine in a cup of coffee is 150 mg, while instant coffee contains approximately 90 mg, tea 75 mg, and cola drinks 60 mg. Caffeine is in a number of the over-the-counter analgesics, including Anacin, Bromo Seltzer, Cope, Empirin Compound, Excedrin, and Vanquish. It is also present in prescription drugs, including propoxyphene (Darvon Compound) and Fiorinal, and it is included in a number of over-the-counter cold preparations. These details are important for the nonmedical clinician as patients may inadvertently accumulate high levels of caffeine, which can produce psychiatric symptoms. Although individual sensitivity varies, symptoms may occur in doses of 200 mg. The symptoms of caffeinism are identical to the classical description of an anxiety episode (Victor et al. 1981). Taking a thorough history of caffeine ingestion is crucial to every evaluation of an anxious patient. It has also been recognized that caffeine withdrawal can be a source of intermittent anxiety (White et al. 1980). Other sympathomimetic stimulants can produce a variety of psychiatric symptoms. Phenylephrine (Neosynephrine), contained in nasal spray, and phenylpropanolomine, found in a multitude of over-the-counter cold preparations, can produce depression, hallucinations, restlessness, and paranoia (Dietz 1981; Escobar and Karno 1982; Snow et al. 1980). Xanthines, such as theophylline, commonly used in the treatment of a variety of pulmonary diseases, can produce significant increases in anxiety and agitation at toxic levels. The patient should have these levels checked, if personality changes take place while on such medication.

Other Commonly Used Drugs

Digitalis toxicity can lead to irritability, agitation, and hallucinations (Greenblatt and Shader 1972; Shear and Sacks 1977–1978). Whenever there is a behavior change in a person on digitalis, the digitalis plasma level should be checked, since mental changes are often the first symptoms of toxicity. Levodopa, and bromocriptine, may lead to a wide variety of symptoms, including depression, mania, hallucinations, and confusion (Goodwin 1972). Finally, cimetidine (Tagamet), used in the treatment of peptic ulcer, has been found to produce confusion, depression, paranoia, and other psychiatric states (Crowder and Pate 1980; Finkelstein and Isselbacher 1978; Weddington et al. 1981).

This abbreviated list of psychiatric side effects of medication is not meant to overwhelm or discourage the nonmedical clinician. It takes a long time to become aware of all the details, and most psychiatrists, except for those who specialize in the practice of medically oriented psychiatry, are unable to maintain an expert level of awareness as to the behavioral consequences of medication. Nevertheless, clinicians should take one step at a time in this area. It is important to create an atmosphere in which the patient feels comfortable in telling someone about any experience, no matter how unusual. Patients should not be made to feel they are "complainers" or "crazy" when reporting possible adverse effects while they are taking the medication. The patient can be the best teacher about the consequences of taking medication, and for the clinician who patiently listens, real knowledge in this area cannot be far off. It is important to keep an open mind and realize that virtually anything is possible while someone is taking a medication, though some side effects are more commonly observed than others. While such effects vary widely in their incidence, they should always be suspected, especially when the time course of the onset of psychiatric symptoms is coincident with a change in medication.

Chemotherapy

Chemotherapy agents are specifically designed poisons used in a carefully controlled program. Since the systemic effect of chemotherapy can be so pervasive, it is no surprise that patients experience a wide variety of generalized secondary consequences such as weakness, fatigue, nausea and vomiting (which are discussed in the following section), malaise, and so on. Many people, but certainly not everyone, feel terrible on chemotherapy. Aside from such nonspecific side effects, certain agents are, in addition, associated with unique psychiatric consequences.

L-Asparaginase can produce confusion, depression, paranoia, or bizarre behavior (Holland et al. 1974). It is an agent currently used mostly for the treatment of acute lymphoblastic leukemia. Vinblastine, used primarily in the treatment of Hodgkin's disease and as part of combination therapy for some testicular tumors, has occasionally been reported to produce depression and anxiety (Peterson and Popkin 1980; Letter 1981). Vincristine (Oncovin) is well known to produce alterations in sensation, muscle function, and autonomic functions (Martin and Compston 1965). The earliest signs of such neuropathic changes include depression of the Achilles tendon reflex at the ankle, followed by tingling sensations in the fingers and toes, leading to weakness, muscle pain, and sensory loss in the extremities. Impairment of the autonomic nervous system can result in constipation or more severe loss of bowel function leading to obstruction. Most symptoms recover following discontinuation of the drug, but the weakness, which may be irreversible, should not be wrongly ascribed to some "psychiatric" condition such as depression or loss of motivation. Recently, some clinicians have supported earlier obversations that this drug may produce depression by alteration of biogenic amines (Silberfarb et al 1983). Vincristine is primarily used as a component of therapy for acute lymphoblastic leukemia, Hodgkin's disease, and non-Hodgkin's lymphomas. It is less commonly used in treatment of breast cancer, some brain tumors, sarcomas, and small-cell carcinoma of the lung.

Among the group of alkylating agents, mechlorethamine (Mustargen) has been reported to produce a toxic encephalopathy that can present with psychiatric symptoms of a wide variety rapidly leading to changes in level of consciousness and delirium (Bethlenfalvay and Bergin 1972; Calabresi and Parks 1975). Similar, but transient, impairment of brain function may result from another alkylating agent cyclophosphamide (Cytoxan), though this is unusual (Tashima 1975).

Among the antimetabolites, there is some suggestion that fluouracil, which does cause the blood brain barrier, can produce delirium (Greenwald 1976) in addition to the ataxia from cerebellar neurotoxicity (Moertel et al. 1964). Methotrexate, when used intrathecally (that is, when administered by spinal tap into the cerebrospinal fluid), occasionally can produce problems such as dementia (Bleyer 1977; Meadows and Evans 1976; Proceedings 1977). One group has reported a significantly higher incidence of anxiety and depression in breast cancer patients receiving cyclophosphamide, methotrexate, and 5-fluorouracil (CMF) compared with patients given melphalan alone (Maguire et al. 1980). A delayed form of encephalopathy may follow several years after successful treatment of leukemia using methotrexate and cranial irradiation in children (Price and Jameson 1975; Rubenstein et al. 1975). Minor neurologic abnormalities such as ataxia or perceptual disorders may also occur as late sequelae (McIntosh et al. 1976).

Given the large number of chemotherapeutic agents available and their pervasive systemic effects, it is somewhat incredible that the CNS alterations leading to loss of cognitive ability or the development of psychiatric systems are so few! It has been very difficult to sort out direct toxic drug effects from some of the indirect effects on the CNS that are secondary to altered function of major organs such as lungs, liver, or kidney. As discussed in chapter 4, there is also evidence that many malignancies produce substances that can drastically alter the body's chemical balance. For example, a high percentage of lung cancer patients produce hormonal substances that have metabolic effects on calcium or sodium concentrations, which then lead to impaired brain function independently of any chemotherapy. Given the prevalence of such chemical imbalances, altered function of major organs due to disease, as well as the presence of many powerful drugs, it is no surprise that there has been recent documentation of a high incidence of cognitive impairment in cancer patients (Oxman and Silberfarb 1980). It appears, however, that such impairments (in memory, concentration, and attention) are probably accounted for by systemic metabolic factors other than the chemotherapy itself (Silberfarb et al. 1980).

Psychiatric Effects of Steroids

Steroids, which include drugs such as prednisone, dexamethasone (Decadron), and methylprednisone (Medrol), are widely used in severely ill patients. They are often included as one component of chemotherapy but are also given chronically or in bursts for such illnesses as systemic lupus erythematosis and severe pulmonary diseases and to control edema associated with brain tumors. Steroids can cause profound psychiatric side effects, which can occur soon after starting the drug, during the time it is being maintained, and when it is being tapered. The effects may include symptoms of depression, irritability, euphoria, or psychosis (Carroll 1981; Ling et al. 1981).

> Evelyn R. is a 67-year-old woman who was admitted to the hospital for her third course of chemotherapy for metastatic breast cancer. The drug regimen includes large doses of steroids. Shortly following admission, she let a nurse know that she changed her mind about further chemotherapy. The staff assumes that she has decided to "give up" on treatment. Some staff quietly express their opinion that she is making the right decision, while others argue that such refusal does not make any sense, especially in light of her basically optimistic personality.

The confrontation with a patient who refuses treatment is pregnant with possibilities. One never knows what is involved, what attitude the patient will have toward discussion, or how the person expects the physician to react. In the "old days," disagreement with a physician about taking a specified treatment was considered tantamount to incompetence. While such an attitude is well behind most of the field, the fact that a psychiatric consultation is often requested for such medical patients may still carry with it the implication that a person is ''crazy'' to refuse any treatment. It is no wonder that many patients are wary when a consultant associated with psychiatry approaches them in such circumstances. Whenever possible, the primary physician should be the one to become involved in trying carefully to understand how the patient's concerns and beliefs have led to a decision to refuse treatment. Only if such basic groundwork has been unproductive, should a psychiatric consultation be considered. The decision by the oncologist or primary physician simply to accept the patient's refusal raises broad social, ethical, and legal contexts discussed further in chapter; most refusals are symptomatic of some other problem in treatment that can usually be addressed within the usual clinical context. Any consultant approaching a patient who is refusing treatment will find it crucial to begin with a personal introduction and something like, ''What's your understanding of why I have been asked to meet with you?'' This opening is important since the consultant will be deprived of his/her position as a problem solver if the patient feels that the hidden agenda is to coerce a changed decision at any price. Many patients will respond by saying, ''You're here because I won't take my medication and you are going to try to talk me into it, I guess.'' The patient must be dissuaded of any such intention. The consultant must clarify, ''Actually, I'm here to try to understand what has been going on in your treatment, what your concerns are, and what would be most helpful to you at this point.'' Once this is clarified, the patient often welcomes the opportunity to put things into perspective because the pathway of events leading to treatment refusal is often strewn with a cascade of complex issues that have left little room for sharing or discussion with others, let along pondering on one's own.

During the initial interview, Mrs. R. stated that her two previous experiences with chemotherapy were unbearable. It is often the tendency for a concerned clinician to empathize with the patient at this point, without further inquiry. However, what the patient needs here is more than just a friend. No clinician should assume that he/she understands such a statement at face value. What does she mean by ''unbearable''? Many of the staff involved with the treatment of patients with cancer have their own ambivalent attitudes toward treatment. This woman went on to elaborate that what frightened her the most about her previous treatments were the horrifying "visions." The psychiatric consultant then elicited that she had in fact said that as much as death frightened her, the likelihood of another such psychotic episode seemed worse and led to her decision to refuse treatment. The consultant was able to reassure her that such "visions" are a well-known side effect of one of the steroid medications, that she was *not* a crazy person, and that this side effect could be recognized in its very early stages and adequately treated.With such reassurance, the patient agreed to treatment. When she began to report an escalating sense of fear, specific treatment (in this case haloperidol) was added to her medications, which resulted in an otherwise unremarkable course and uneventful discharge from the hospital. It is not always so easy to connect psychiatric symptoms to the steroids since it may be very difficult to sort out the effects of brain involvement from the disease from the effects of the drug.

Treatment of Nausea and Vomiting: Medication and Beyond

There is some rationale for discussing nausea and vomiting in a chapter on the psychiatric consequences of cancer and its treatment. Nausea and vomiting are among the most common and most distressing problems for the cancer patient and their control is essential for the patient's well-being and survival (Frytak and Moertel 1981). Both radiation therapy and certain drugs induce vomiting by affecting nerves that have input into the anatomic "vomiting center" located in the brain stem. Other drugs induce vomiting by effects on a part of the brain known as the "chemoreceptor trigger zone." However, there are many other neuronal pathways that have input into this zone and thereby induce vomiting. Therefore, the situation is more complex and involves an interplay of physical and psychological factors which, once understood, can be exploited for therapeutic gain.

The treatment of nausea and vomiting obviously depends first on identification and correction of the underlying medical cause whenever possible. Sometimes, however, nausea and vomiting continue to be a major problem despite scrupulous attention to the contributing medical factors. In such circumstances, awareness of several basic psychological principles of learning theory can lead to some simple interventions that often make the world of difference for the patient.

Nausea and Vomiting as a Conditioned Response

Many cancer chemotherapy drugs cause nausea and vomiting beginning one to two hours after medication injection and persisting for two to 24 hours. About 20% of patients will volunteer that they experience nausea even as they enter the clinic or office, before any treatment is given (Morrow 1982). Such a phenomenon is often dismissed as anticipatory anxiety, "nerves," or a reflection of some underlying psychological aversion to treatment. However, it is often more useful to view such nausea and vomiting as a conditioned response (Nesse et al. 1980).

The classical model for producing such conditioning is based on Pavlov's original and well-known experiment in which he conditioned a dog to salivate at the sound of a bell. In that situation, the dog is first exposed to food to elicit salivation. The food is an unconditioned stimulus and the salivation is an unconditioned response. Such a relationship is patterned into our CNS and is a basic part of our behavioral repertoire which no one has to learn; hence it is "unconditioned."

Unconditioned *Unconditioned*
stimulus (UCS) *response (UCR)*
Food   ⇨   Salivation

To train the dog, Pavlov began to ring a bell every time the dog was presented with food. He therefore "paired" an unconditioned stimulus (food) with another stimulus (the bell) that he wished to condition.

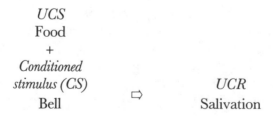

Finally, once associative pathways are established in the nervous system as a result of the pairing process, the CS alone (the bell) is sufficient to induce the response of salivation.

Conditioned		*Conditioned*
stimulus (CS)	⇨	*response (CR)*
Bell		Salivation

An identical model has been proposed to explain a variety of situations in which patients experience nausea and vomiting. In such cases, since the chemotherapy agent can produce nausea and vomiting on a straightforward neurological basis, it is an example of unconditioned stimulus (UCS) producing an unconditioned response (UCR) of nausea and vomiting.

Unconditioned		*Unconditioned*
stimulus (UCS)	⇨	*response (UCR)*
Chemotherapy		Nausea and vomiting

The opportunity for "pairing" the UCS with a variety of other stimuli is ubiquitous and seems almost unavoidable. Certainly visual or olfactory stimuli in the clinic setting may become paired and therefore "conditioned" to produce nausea and vomiting on their own.

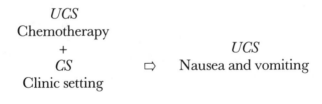

UCS		
Chemotherapy		
+		*UCS*
CS	⇨	Nausea and vomiting
Clinic setting		

| *CS* | | *CR* |
| Clinic setting alone | ⇨ | Nausea and vomiting |

More subtly, some image or thought of the clinic may in itself serve as a conditioned stimulus. It should be emphasized that such events occur commonly in everyday nonmedical settings, as can be attested to by anyone who has become nauseated by seeing or smelling some food or beverage that had previously led to vomiting because of food poisoning.

Awareness of this learning model leads to important treatment implications since it implies that a behavioral intervention will be effective. In the case of the patient who has become conditioned to vomit upon entering the clinic, a brief training program in relaxation, combined with some "counterconditioning," can be dramatic and quickly effective (Morrow and Morrell, 1982; Nesse, et al. 1980). Counterconditioning is accomplished by teaching the patient to relax and "pairing" some other more pleasant image with the clinic setting to create a stimulus situation that is incompatible with nausea and vomiting. Counterconditioning may be accompanied by learning a simple relaxation method that can be practiced in the setting normally leading to the nausea and vomiting. At other times, it may be necessary to combine relaxation with visualization of pleasant images or with hypnotic suggestion. (Burish and Lyles, 1979). LaBaw et al. (1975) reported a decrease in chemotherapy-associated nausea vomiting by training children in self-hypnosis. In any case, this learning-theory-based treatment model seems to be underutilized. The anorexia that develops to specific foods during a course of chemotherapy may also represent a conditioned phenomenon (Bernstein and Sigmundi 1980). Behavioral techniques are not suggested as a substitute for medication but as an adjunct or alternative to be considered. As another benefit, those patients who are exposed to this treatment modality often develop an increased sense of well-being and self-mastery because of their increased ability to calm themselves (Weisman and Sobel 1979). One of the beauties of such approaches is that they seem to be quite cost-effective since they are often successful given one or two sessions with some home follow-up training by the patient (Burish and Lyles, 1981).

Medication for Nausea and Vomiting

Nausea and vomiting are not always a direct side effect of the illness or its treatment, or even a conditioned phenomenon. At times, they represent a psychological response to the illness (Chang 1981). The nonspecific beneficial effects of family and caring relationship with the anxious patient and eliciting of issues of concern should not be underestimated. The semistructured interview included in the appendix may be a useful framework for such work with the patient. Anxiety associated with treatment can be effectively dealt with in patients by self-regulatory relaxation techniques (Goldberg 1982).

There are, of course, a variety of medications used to combat nausea and vomiting. The most widely used, by far, belong to the class of drugs known as the phenothiazines, of which prochlorperazine (Compazine) is the most popular. This group of drugs is well absorbed orally and works directly to suppress the chemoreceptor trigger zone in the brain stem. Unfortunately, it is effective only for mild degrees of nausea and vomiting and is inadequate for the distress associated with such agents as cisplatin, for example. Incidentally, Compazine is available in an extended-release spansule which, although significantly more costly, has no decided advantage over its less expansive oral tablet counterpart. It is also available as a rectal suppository, which is useful for patients in the home setting when vomiting would render an oral agent ineffective. Other phenothiazines such as chlorpromazine (Thorazine), perphenazine (Trilafon), and trifluoperazine (Stelazine), are also effective antiemetics and may have fewer side effects. Investigation of the antiemetic effects of haloperidol (Haldol) are underway (Neidhart et al. 1980).

Other antiemetic agents are available, though decisive data to confirm their efficacy are lacking. Neither trimethobenzamide (Tigan) nor benzquinamide hydrochloride (Emetecon) have been demonstrated to be superior to placebo in cancer patients (Moertel and Reitemeier 1969; Purkis 1965). Anecdotal reports of the efficacy of marijuana in reducing chemotherapy-associated nausea and vomiting have led to experiments confirming that THC (tetrahydrocannabinol, the presumed active ingredient in marijuana) is an extremely effective antiemetic in some situations (Sallan et al. 1980). It has been shown to be effective in preventing nausea and vomiting associated with high-dose methotrexate therapy, but not for combination treatment with cyclophosphamide and doxorubicin hydrochloride (Chang et al. 1979). In a study comparing prochlorperazine (Compazine) and THC for a group of over 100 cancer patients receiving chemotherapy (Frytak et al. 1979), the two drugs performed about equally in preventing nausea and vomiting; however, there were more side effects in the THC group, including hallucinations and other disquieting symptoms. One group reports 36% more hallucinations for patients receiving THC at antiemetic doses (Kluin-Nelreman et al. 1979). A more optimistic review of the literature notes that THC can be a superior antiemetic and that, at moderate doses, it has manageable side effects consisting mostly of somnolence, conjunctivitis, and tachycardias (Poster et al. 1981). At present, it appears that THC has some place in the drug armamentarium and may be best suited for patients who feel comfortable talking such a drug and who have proved resistent to more conventional treatment. However, general availability of THC may be a problem for many patients. Finally, metoclopramide (Reglan) is a drug currently receiving attention because of its potential for preventing the particularly disabling nausea and vomiting associated with cisplatin therapy (Shulze-Delricu 1981).

The Use of Tranquilizers in Cancer Patients

Aside from antiemetics such as prochlorperazine (Compazine), sedative-hypnotics are the most widely prescribed psychotropic medications for cancer patients (Derogatis, et al. 1979). This group includes drugs such as diazepam (Valium) and flurazepam (Dalmane). The clinician should be aware of a number of issues pertinent to this drug group (Goldberg 1982). First of all, diazepam (Valium) prescribing has become a highly politicized issue. Following a major journalistic "exposé" of Valium overprescribing, overuse, and addictive potential on CBS "60 Minutes," the public became more aware of our exaggerated societal dependence on chemical tranquilizers and their associated dangers. An anti-Valium backlash left many prescribing physicians feeling as if they were criminals, and many patients who were taking the drug for valid reasons feeling as if they were dope addicts. It is to be hoped that such an antidrug backlash has served as a corrective measure for earlier practices and people can begin to consider the appropriate use of this medication. Drugs such as Valium are best used in the short term to assist in coping with excessively stressful circumstances. Used for relatively brief periods of time, weeks to a few months, for example, in moderate doses, such drugs are not addicting, and create no fundamental dangers for the user. Disabling anxiety, for its own part, can claim no redeeming attributes. In addition, there is no evidence that the moderate use of the tranquilizer impairs the ability of a person psychologically to interpret important experiences.

For the vast majority of people who are given Valium in the context of major medical illness, addiction and dependence are not the main issues to be concerned about. The most insidious and destructive effects of such drugs have to do with producing a general dulling of mental processes and alertness, leading to an overall lower level of physical and mental function than the patient is truly capable of. Diazepam (Valium), chlordiazepoxide (Librium), and clorazepate (Tranxene) stay in the body for long periods of time before they are fully metabolized and, therefore, may tend to accumulate to toxic levels over time. Alternatives, such as lorazepam (Ativan), oxazepam (Serax), and alprazolam (Xanax), which are just as effective in reducing anxiety, are not associated with such cumulative potential and are often a better choice.

Roberta is a 56-year-old, married mother of three who had been working as an insurance adjuster until her recent hospital readmission for back pain. She had a total abdominal hysterectomy two years before for an early stage of uterine cancer. Her back pain had been present for several months before this admission and necessitated her absence from work, an adjustment she found particularly difficult given her action-oriented-personality style. Unable to stay in bed and relax, she became more and more wound up and was placed on diazepam (Valium), 5 mg three times a day, by her physician, who aftersome initial negative screening X-rays, decided to take a conservative approach in her treatment. Her husband reported that she had been having increasingly frequent crying spells over the week before admission and had become impossible to talk to, at first because of her irritability, and then because of her withdrawal. A psychiatric consultation was requested to help this patient deal with her "psychological adjustment to her medical condition" and make her more cooperative with the necessary diagnostic process. During the initial interview, the consultant found this patient morose, slow to respond to questions, and somewhat confused about the details of her symptoms over the previous few months. She was generally opposed to large amounts of pain medication and had taken only two aspirin tablets four times a day despite prescriptions by her physician for oxycodone (Percodan), an orally taken narcotic. The consultant, after careful testing of her memory, orientation, and intellectual functioning, felt that the amount of diazepam (Valium) was a major factor contributing to her psychological demise since its accumulation could readily lead to her mental dulling and sedation, which in themselves were difficult for this patient to tolerate. At his recommendation, the Valium was discontinued and the workup proceeded. Within two days, the patient's mood brightened, she became more socially interactive, and she stated that it was the first time she felt like herself since starting the Valium weeks before.

Clinicians working with patients who are on such medication must be aware of their potential to produce depressing effects and should not be afraid to raise the issue of having the dose reduced or the medication changed to one of the group with a shorter half-life (half-life being the time it takes for the body to metabolize 50% of the drug taken). Overall, the benzodiazepines have little toxicity and few consistent unwanted effects. Their most common adverse effects involve the CNS and produce depression, muscle weakness, ataxia, difficulty in speaking, dizziness, sleepiness, and confusion. There is some question as to whether or not benzodiazepines release hostility and rage reactions in some people (Di-Mascio et al. 1970; Karch 1979). Certainly clinicians may notice that some patients started on benzodiazepines become more agitated and aggressive. In such instances, which probably represent some type of disinhibition phenomenon, the patient can be switched to oxazepam (Serax), which may have a lower reported incidence to this effect (Kochansky et al. 1975, 1977). In addition to the release of hostility, chlordiazepoxide (Librium) may have a paradoxical stimulating effect in some patients (Hall and Jaffe 1972). In others, it may produce or increase depressive symptomology (Ryan et al. 1978). Drugs such as barbiturates, glutethimide (Doriden), ethchlorvynol (Placidyl), meprobamate (Miltown), or methaqualone (Quaaludes) have a much higher addictive potential, create a more rapid onset of tolerance with a need to escalate the dose, and have a narrower safe dosage range with a greater tendency to cause toxic symptoms.

When a sleeping pill is warranted, there are a number of possibilities. Flurazepam (Dalmane) has been marketed most successfully and is the most widely used drug in this category in recent years. However, it is not well appreciated that the accumulation of its active metabolite can at times lead to toxic effects. In any patient, especially in older patients or those with liver impairment, such prolongation of drug activity is even more exaggerated and frequently leads to episodes of confusion or impaired psychomotor performance. Recently two new drugs in this group, temazepam (Restoril), and triazolam (Halcion) been marketed. Because their half-lives are around ten hours and three hours respectively, they are claimed to be more sensible choices for sleep, and are said to produce less daytime hangover and few, if any, cumulative effects. Therefore, it is likely that these drugs will capture a significant portion of the market over the next year or so. They appear to be about as effective as other available choices. A complete discussion of the issues involved in determining the efficacy of hypnotics goes beyond the scope of this chapter. Suffice it to say that no hypnotic has been demonstrated to be effective beyond a fairly limited period of time (approximately one month) and that long-term chronic use is of questionable value.

Hypnotics are not a solution for most of the conditions that interfere with sleep in cancer patients. One of the most common in patients with life-threatening illness is inadequately treated pain, which is discussed separately in chapter 6. Another problem that causes sleep impairment is depression, which, as discussed in chapter 4, should be treated with an antidepressant rather than a hypnotic.

References

ABELSON, H. I., AND FISHBURNE, P. M.: Nonmedical use of psychoactive substances: 1975–76. Nationwide study among youth and adults. Response Analysis Corp., Princeton, N.J., 1976.

ABROMOWICZ, M. (Ed.): Drugs that cause psychiatric symptoms. *Med. Letter* 23 (1981): 9–12.

BERNSTEIN, I. L., AND SIGMUNDI, R. A.: Tumor anorexia: A learned food aversion? *Science* 209 (1980): 416–418.

BETHLENFALVAY, N. C., AND BERGIN, J. J.: Severe cerebral toxicity after intravenous nitrogen mustard therapy. *Cancer* 29 (1972): 366.

BLACKWELL, B.: Patient compliance. *N. Engl. J. Med.* 289 (1975): 249–252.

BLEYER, W. A.: Methotrexate: Clinical pharmacology, current status, and therapeutic guidelines. *Cancer Treat. Rev.* 4 (1977): 87.

BURISH, T. G., AND LYLES, J. N.: Effectiveness of relaxation training in reducing adverse reactions to cancer chemotherapy. *J. Behav. Med.* 4 (1981): 65–78.

————: Effectiveness of relaxation training in reducing the aversiveness of chemotherapy in the treatment of cancer. *J. Behav. Ther. Exp. Psychiatry* 10 (1979): 357–361.

Byck, R.: Psychologic factors in drug administration. In *Clinical pharmacology*, 2nd ed. K. L. Melmon, H. F. Morelli, Eds. New York: Macmillan, 1978, chap. 4.

Calabresi, P., Parks, R. E., Jr.: In L. S. Goodman and A. Gilman (Eds.), *The pharmacological basis of therapeutics*, 5th ed. New York: Macmillan, 1975, p. 1254.

Carroll, B. J.: Psychiatric disorders and steroids. E. Usdin, D. A. Hamburg, and J. D. Barchas (Eds.), In *Neuroregulators and Psychiatric Disorders*. Oxford: Oxford University Press, 1977, chapt. 31.

Cassileth, B. R.: After laetrile, what? *N. Engl. J. Med.* 301 (1982): 1482–1484.

Chang, A., Shiling, D., Stillman, R., Goldberg, N., Steipp, C., Barotsky, I., Simon, R., and Rosenberg, S.: Delta-9-tetrahydrocannabinol as an antiemetic in cancer patients receiving high-dose methotrexate. *Ann. Intern. Med.* 91 (1979): 819–824.

Chang, J. C.: Nausea and vomiting in cancer patients: An expression of psychological mechanisms? *Psychosomatics* 22 (1981): 707–709.

Crowder, M. K., and Pate, J. K.: A case report of cimetidine-induced depressive syndrome. *Am. J. Psychiatry* 137 (1980): 11.

Davidson, J. R. T., Raft, D., Lewis, B. F., and Gebhardt, M.: Psychotropic drugs on general medical and surgical wards of a teaching hospital. *Arch. Gen. Psychiatry* 32 (1975): 507–511.

Derogatis, L. R., Feldstein, M., Morrow, G., et al.: A survey of psychotropic drugs prescriptions in an oncology population. *Cancer* 44 (1979): 1919–1929.

Dietz, A. J.: Amphetamine-like reactions to phenylpropanolamine. *JAMA* 245 (1981): 601–602.

DiMascio, A., Shader, R. I., and Giller, D. R.: Behavioral toxicity. Part III: Perceptual-cognitive functions: Part IV: Emotional- (mood) states. In R. I. Shader, and A. DiMascio (Eds.), *Psychotropic drug side effects*. Baltimore: Williams & Wilkins, 1970, pp. 132–141.

Escobar, J. I., and Karno, M.: Chronic hallucinosis from nasal drops. *JAMA* 247 (1982): 1859–1860.

Finkelstein, W., and Isselbacher, K. J.: Drug therapy: Cimetidine. *N. Engl. J. Med.* 299 (1978): 992–996.

Franks, R. D., and Richter, A. J.: Schizophrenia-like psychosis associated with anticonvulsant toxicity. *Am. J. Psychiatry* 136 (1979): 973.

FRYTAK, S., AND MOERTEL, C. G.: Management of nausea and vomiting in the cancer patient. *JAMA* 245 (1981): 393–396.

FRYTAK, S., MOERTEL, C. G., O'FALLON, J. R., ET AL.: Delta-9-tetrahydrocannabinol as an antiemetic for patients receiving cancer cheomotherapy. *Ann. Intern. Med.* 91 (1979): 825–830.

GOLDBERG, R. J.: Anxiety reduction by self-regulation: Theory, practice, and evaluation. *Ann. Intern. Med.* 96 (1982): 483–487.

_____: Benzodiazepines. In R. J. Goldberg (Ed.), *Anxiety: A guide to biobehavioral diagnosis and therapy for physicians and mental health clinicians.* Garden City, N. Y.: Medical Examination Publishing Co. 1982.

GOLDSTEIN, A., AND KAIZER, S.: Psychotropic effects of caffeine in man, III. *Clin. Pharmacol. Ther.* 10 (1969): 477–488.

GOODWIN, F. K.: Behavioral effects of L-dopa in man. In R. I. Shader (Ed.), *Psychiatric complications of medical drugs.* New York: Raven Press, 1972, chap. 6.

GREENBLATT, D. J., AND SHADER, R. I.: Digitalis toxicity. In R. I. Shader (Ed.), *Psychiatric complications of medical drugs.* New York: Raven Press, 1972, chap. 2.

GREENWALD, E. S.: Organic mental changes with fluorouvacil therapy. *JAMA*: 235 (1976): 248–249.

HALL, R. C. W., FEINSILVER, D. L., AND HOLT, R. E.: Anticholinergic psychosis: Differential diagnosis and management. *Psychosomatics* 22 (1981): 581–587.

HALL, R. W. C., AND JAFFE, J. R.: Aberrant response to diazepam: A new syndrome. *Am. J. Psychiatry* 126 (1972): 738–742.

HOLLAND, J., FASANELLO, S., AND OHNUMA, T.: Psychiatric symptoms associated with L-asparaginase administration. *J. Psychiatr. Res.* 10 (1974): 113–150.

JOHNSON, A. L., HOLLISTER, L. E., AND BERGER, P. A.: The anticholinergic intoxication syndrome: Diagnosis and treatment. *J. Clin. Psychiatry* 42 (1981): 313–317.

KARCH, F. E.: Rage reaction associated with clorazepate dipotassium. *Ann. Intern. Med.* 91 (1979): 61–62.

KLUIN-NELEMAN, J. C., NELEMAN, F. A., MEUWISSEN, O. J. A. T., ET AL.: Delta-9-tetrahydrocannabinol (THC) as an antiemetic in patients treated with cancer chemotherapy: A double-blind crossover trial against placebo. *Vet. Human Toxicol.* 21 (1979): 338–340.

KOCHANSKY, G. E., SALZMAN, C., SHADER, R. I., ET AL.: Effects of chlordiazepoxide and oxazepam administration on verbal hostility. *Arch. Gen. Psychiatry* 34 (1977): 1457–1459.

————: The differential effects of chlordiazepoxide and oxazepam on hostility in a small group setting. *Am. J. Psychiatry* 132 (1975): 861–863.

LaBaw, W., Holton, C., Tewell, K., and Eccles, D.: The use of self-hypnosis by children with cancer. *Am. J. Clin. Hypn.* 17 (1975): 233–238.

Ling, M. H. M., Perry, P. J., and Tsuang, M. T.: Side effects of corticosteroid therapy. *Arch. Gen. Psychiatry* 38 (1981): 471–477.

Loftus, E. F., and Fries, J. F.: Informed consent may be hazardous to health. *Science* 204 (1979): 11.

Maguire, G. P., Tait, A., Brooke, M., et al.: Psychiatric morbidity and physical toxicity associated with adjuvant chemotherapy after mastectomy. *Br. Med. J.* 281 (1980): 1179–1180.

Martin, J., and Compston, N.: Vincristine sulfate in the treatment of lymphoma and leukemia. *Lancet* 2 (1965): 1080.

Meadows, A. T., and Evans, A. E.: Effects of chemotherapy on the central nervous system. *Cancer* 37 (Feb. 1976): 1079–1085, suppl.

Moertel, C. G., and Reitemeier, R. J.: Advanced gastrointestinal cancer/clinical management and chemotherapy. New York: Harper & Row, 1969, p. 38.

Moertel, C. G., Reitemeier, R. J., Bolton, C. F., et al.: Cerebellar ataxia associated with fluorinated pyrimidine therapy. *Cancer. Chemother. Rep.* 41 (1964): 15–18.

Morrow, G. R.: Prevalence and correlates of anticipatory nausea and vomiting in chemotherapy patients. *J. Nat. Cancer Inst.* 68 (1982): 585–588.

Morrow, G. R., and Morrell, C.: Behavioral treatment for the anticipatory nausea and vomiting induced by cancer chemotherapy. *N. Engl. J. Med.* 307 (1982): 1476–1480.

Neidhart, J., Gagen, M., and Metz, E.: Haldol as an effective antiemetic for platinum and mustard induced vomiting when other agents fail. *Proc. ACO-AACR* 21 (1980): 365.

Nesse, R. M., Carli, T., Curtis, G. C., and Kleinman, P. D.: Pretreatment nausea in cancer chemotherapy: A conditioned response? *Psychosom. Med.* 42 (1980): 33–36.

Oxman, T. E., and Silberfarb, P. M.: Serial cognitive testing in cancer patients receiving chemotherapy. *Am. J. Psychiatry* 137 (1980): 1263–1265.

Paykel, E. S., Pleminger, R., and Watson, J. P.: Psychiatric side effects of antihypertensive drugs other than reserpine. *J. Clin. Psychopharmacol.* 2 (1982), 1: 14–39.

PETERSON, L. G., AND POPKIN, M. K.: Neuropsychiatric effects of chemotherapeutic agents for cancer. *Psychosom.* 21: 141–153, 1980.

POSTER, D. S., PENTA, J. S., BRUNO, S., AND MACDONALD, J. S.: Delta-9-tetrahydrocannabinol in clinical oncology. *JAMA* 245 (1981): 2047–2051.

Proceedings of the workshop on antimetabolites and the central nervous system. *Cancer Treat. Rep.* 61 (1977): 505.

PURKIS, I. E.: The action of thiethylperazine (torecan), a new antiemetic compared with perphenazine (Trilafon), trimethobenzamide (Tigan), and a placebo in the suppression of postanesthetic nausea and vomiting. *Can. Anaesth. Soc. J.* 12 (1965): 595–607.

RIVINUS, TIM.: Psychiatric effects of anticonvulsant regimens. *J. Clin. Psychopharmacol.* 2 (1982): 165–192.

RYAN, H. F., MERRILL, F. B., SCOTT, G. E., ET AL.: Increase in suicidal thoughts and tendencies. Association with diazepam therapy. *JAMA* 203 (1968): 1137–1139.

SALLAN, S. E., CRONIC, C., ZELEN, M., ET AL.: Antiemetics in patients receiving chemotherapy for cancer. *N. Engl. J. Med.* 302 (1980): 135–138.

SALZMAN, C.: Psychotropic drugs use and polypharmacy in a general hospital. *Gen. Hosp. Psychiatry* 3 (1981): 1–9.

SCHULZE-DELRIEU, K.: Metoclopramide. *N. Engl. J. Med.* 305 (1981): 28–33.

SILBERFARB, P. M., PHILIBERT, D., AND LEVINE, P. M.: Psychosocial aspects of neoplastic disease: II. Affective and cognitive effects of chemotherapy in cancer patients. *Am. J. Psychiatry* 137 (1980): 597–601.

SILBERFARB, P. M., HOLLAND, J. C. B., ANBAR, D., ET AL.: Psychological response of patients receiving two drug regimens for lung carcinoma. *Am. J. Psychiatry* 140 (1983): 110–111.

SHEAR, M. K., AND SACKS, M.: Digitalis delirium: Psychiatric considerations. *Int. J. Psychiatry Med.* 8 (1977–1978): 371–380.

SNOW, S. S., ET AL.: Nasal spray addiction and psychosis. A case report. *Br. J. Psychiatry* 136 (1980): 297.

TASHIMA, C. K.: Immediate cerebral symptoms during rapid intravenous administration of cyclophosophamide (NLC-26271). *Cancer Chemother. Rep. Part I* 59 (1975): 441.

TOLLEFSON, G.: Psychiatric implications of anticonvulsant drugs. *J. Clin. Psychiatry* 41 (1980): 295.

VICTOR, B. S., LUBETSKY, M., AND GREDEN, J. F.: Somatic manifestations of caffeinism. *J. Clin. Psychiatry* 42 (1981): 185–188.

WEDDINGTON, W. W., MUELLING, A. E., MOOSA, H. H., ET AL.: Cimetidine toxic reactions masquerading as delirium tremens. *JAMA* 245 (1981): 1058–1059.

WEISMAN, A. D., AND SOBEL, H. J.: Coping with cancer through self instruction: A hypothesis. *J. Human Stress* 5 (1979): 3–8.

WHITE, B. C., ET AL.: Anxiety and muscle tension as consequences of caffeine withdrawal. *Science* 209 (1980): 1547–1548.

CHAPTER 6

Pain

FOR PATIENTS ATTEMPTING to make some adjustment to cancer, the specter of chronic, unremitting pain is certainly the most disturbing and unwanted visitor. The idea that cancer brings with it unavoidable protracted agony seems to be part of the folk medicine heritage of our times. Despite advances in disease treatment and pain control, people seem to be surprised and somewhat skeptical when they are clearly told that pain is not inevitable and that successful pain control is achievable in virtually every patient. And despite such potential success, the experience of many patients and their families is that pain control is less than satisfactory. A rapid survey of advanced cancer patients in many settings reveals that pain remains one of the salient issues for patients, families, physicians, and nursing staff. For all those concerned about or currently involved with pain, this chapter is intended to reveal the biased attitudes and gaps in knowledge that commonly interfere with optimal pain management.

Pain is a private experience. There is no machine or instrument that can quantify the amount of pain that someone feels. Pain is a complex product spawned by neurophysiologic processes modified by the personality, influenced by memories, fantasies, and cultural traditions, and finally expressed in behaviors that connect the patient, family, and health care providers (Merskey and Spear 1967). Pain serves an important signaling function for the organism and often leads to recognition of some underlying disease that can be surgically cut out or medically healed. However, despite the available technology, pain often remains inadequately treated, at times because of underlying physician or patient attitudes and sometimes because of personality conflict between the patient and provider. Despite the fact that both the patient and physician want pain control there are a number of situations in which pain typically remains a problem: (a) After surgery, when the patient complains of excessive pain, the physician is often overly judicious about the prescription of narcotics and insists that the patient get no more "shots," prescribing only a lower (and often inadequate) dose of oral analgesics. (b) When the etiology of pain has not been resolved by diagnostic and therapeutic medical procedures, pain continues. When physicians have the impression that "it shouldn't be there anymore," or at least that "there is no reason for the pain to be that bad," the symptom may go untreated. (c) When pain is not relieved by doses of medication that work for most people, it is therefore assumed to represent some "psychological problem." Because "nothing else seemed to work," the patient in pain may be given a placebo injection of saline solution. When the patient reports "feeling a little better," everyone concludes that pain is "not real." (d) When there is a chronic cause for pain the physician (or patient) feels concerned about avoiding "addiction."

The single most common factor behind these problems of unrelieved severe pain is the underutilization of adequate amounts of analgesic medication (Marks and Sachar 1973). Before going into complex explanations involving personality and social factors, many pain problems can be eliminated simply by increasing the medication dose. What keeps this from happening? The answer seems to emerge from the twin roots of ignorance and moral bias. Many physicians lack sufficient knowledge about the pharmacology of analgesics and many providers, patients, and family members hold a moral bias against taking medication, considering it an unacceptable sign of weakness. It is most difficult to address the deep-seated cultural attitude that putting up with pain is a sign of moral strength and that excessive reliance on "drugs" signals a sign of lack of moral fiber to be condemned. Such staunchly self-reliant quasi-religious fervor emerges most regularly around the issue of addiction. Usually this issue is raised when the physician begins to feel uncomfortable about meeting the patient's escalating demands for medication. At other times, it may be the patient's own distorted sense of what addiction involves that interferes with accepting reasonable treatment.

Sorting out the meaning of addiction may help to deal with this perceived threat more realistically. The term addiction contains three components that must be clearly distinguished. One aspect of addiction refers to *physical tolerance*, an inevitable consequence of the daily use of narcotic analgesics. With repeated exposure, the nervous system adapts to the presence of narcotics, and thus, after awhile, a higher dose is required to obtain the same effect. Tolerance develops not only to the analgesic effects of the medication but also to some of the side effects, such as sedation and depression of respiratory function. A second aspect usually considered part of addiction refers to *physical dependence*, which results from the fact that the nervous system "gets used to" the presence of a drug and creates withdrawal symptoms when the drug dose is lowered or discontinued. Both physical tolerance and dependence are predictable and acceptable aspects of continuous narcotic analgesia and should not be considered reasons to deter the patient from receiving adequate amounts of analgesia, the family from encouraging adequate drug usage, or the physician from prescribing enough medication. Unfortunately, the specter of the narcotic "addict," with its negative connotations, continues to haunt medical practice and often leads to unnecessary suffering. In fact, neither of the two factors, physical dependence or tolerance, is what makes the narcotic "addict" a disreputable, antisocial character. It is the third feature within the term addiction, *drug craving*, a global psychological preoccupation with obtaining the using drugs, that leads to the socially unacceptable behaviors of the "street addict." It is crucial for the patient, family, and physician to bear in mind that such an unfortunate behavioral outcome is rarely encountered in medical patients who are given even high doses of narcotics under medical supervision. Contrary to some opinions, people are able to function at high intellectual and social levels for long periods of time on very high doses of narcotics. High-dose narcotics, in themselves, do not subvert or pervert the patient. Although there seem to be little definitive data in this area, it has been estimated by several authorities that iatrogenic addiction (i.e., the creation of compulsive drug-seeking behaviors in medical patients) occurs in less than 1% of patients and should not be a consideration in the denial of adequate pain relief (Miller and Jick 1978; Porter and Jick 1980). While it should be needless to state, terminal patients should be provided as much analgesia as required. Such situations are becoming rare, but the fear of creating addiction sometimes keeps a physician from providing high-dose narcotics even to a patient who is expected to die within weeks.

Patients should be able to make some decisions about pain medication without the unnecessary pejorative distortions associated with the addiction fears that haunt our society. Patients are entitled to large amounts of narcotics if that is what it takes to control pain. At the same time, they are entitled to receive medication in a way that maximizes their overall goals of adjustment. For example, many people do not wish to be excessively sedated or out of touch with those around them. Patients with such concerns need not deprive themselves of adequate analgesia since, as this chapter will demonstrate, many modifications of drug regimens are available that can maximize pain relief and minimize secondary disabilities. Achieving such custom-tailored drug regimens requires close collaboration of the patient with a nurse or physician knowledgeable in this area. We believe that the nurse-clinical specialist can play a special role in the area of monitoring medication regimens. (Also see chapter 8.) The nurse's position is structured to allow the time to make the daily and often multiple visits needed to monitor response to analgesics. After all, the initial orders can only be best guesses of what eventually will help the patient. More important, the nurse-clinical specialist has the advantage of having better access to the nursing system and the hospital, which are so crucial in delivering the medication and interacting with the patient. It has also been demonstrated in an outpatient setting that home visits by a nurse practitioner can play an important role in improving pain control in patients in advanced stages of cancer (McKegney et al. 1981). The nurse–patient interaction can be the key factor in pain treatment problems, as described in the following section on psychosocial dysfunction and pain management.

Some review of available analgesics and the problems typically encountered with them is in order, though this chapter does not pretend to provide a comprehensive sourcebook of pharmacology. Rather, it presents the providers and patient (or family) with information to help them effectively to negotiate in the medical care system. Ultimately, however, most patients and families will not know as much as the physician and cannot approach the problem by trying to become the authority.

Nurses, social workers, psychologists, and psychiatrists sometimes find themselves in a frustrating situation in which, while they may know enough about issues in pain management to feel that the prescribing physician needs to change the orders, they may not consider themselves to be in position to effect the change. It is not unusual to find, for example, visiting nurses frustrated by physicians who are curt on the telephone or social workers who are told in so many words that they have no business being involved in the medical care of the patient. Indignation is not an effective strategy, and only serves to widen the gap between the primary physician or the medical specialist and the psychosocial consultant. It is probably true that the more knowledgeable and articulate the professional feels, the greater the likelihood of colleague recognition. However, taking on a resistant position is rarely a useful strategy. It is more effective to enlist patients as advocates for their own treatment. If the patient is not in a position to function as an effective advocate, some family member or close friend involved in the treatment may be so. Use of such support to influence the physician has a number of advantages. It keeps psychosocial consultants from getting into a nonproductive adversarial position with the primary physician. It helps to develop a sense of efficacy on behalf of the patient or support person. Involving the support person eliminates the iatrogenic splitting of that person away from the patient by intervening professionally when it really may not be necessary to do so. The support persons are often frustrated in their quest for ways to feel they can do something, and by learning how to be more effective advocates for the patient, they can be made to feel better about their own plight. The principle of intervention here is to become an educator for the patients or support persons, assisting them to become more effective participants in the treatment process. This principle is discussed in greater detail in the part on social support in chapter 3. Increased knowledge in this area will be useful for creating a dialogue with physicians and fostering better collaboration to bring relief of suffering.

A Review of Analgesic Medication

A thorough knowledge of the pharmacology of analgesics and their application combines both science and craft. Such skills are not easily conveyed in a summary or mastered by a review course.

Yet the following principles are basic to any pain management program. Analgesics alone are not the preferred approach to all pain, but should, of course, be integrated within a comprehensive treatment program aimed at the underlying disease process in the context of a psychological approach to the patient that takes individual needs into account.

The psychology of prescribing is an important, and often overlooked, part of medical care. The prescription is never written or taken in a vacuum, but always occurs in the context of a relationship, a psychological set, and a sociocultural matrix.

Lack of response to medication is frequently attributable to noncompliance. When effective medication such as an analgesic is partially mediated by emotion and anxiety, the psychological state of the patient can be an especially important factor in response. If there seems to be a problem with any medication, one factor to consider is whether or not the patient has heard of the medication before, and if so, what the patient has heard. For example, a patient may have heard that some medication was linked with a death—"My uncle took that for a week before he died," or with an adverse side effect—"A friend in my club took that and said she felt dizzy and strange." Such distortions can sometimes be dealt with on a rational level, though at other times it may be important to change the medication if it makes the patient too uncomfortable to use it.

The next important psychological factor in prescribing analgesics is to impart to the patient a sense of availability, receptiveness, and responsiveness. A patient who has been on a variety of medications with mixed effects may not trust a new consultant to be any more effective. Underlying resentments about continued pain will carry over to the new consultant despite the patient's wish for things to be better. To enlist the patient as an ally, it is important to say something to the effect that:

> You have been on quite a number of medications for your pain and it seems that things have been continuing to be a problem. I am going to eliminate a lot of confusion that has been taking place and will coordinate your medication orders to make them both simpler and more effective. Most important, I will work with you to custom tailor the medication to your unique needs. I will count on you to let me know how things are going and you can count on me to listen to make appropriate changes.

This message usually reduces the patient's anxiety significantly and can be an important factor in the patient's response to the new analgesic program.

Analgesics can be broadly divided into two classes: narcotics and nonnarcotics representing two levels of pain relief.

Nonnarcotic Analgesics

The nonnarcotic analgesics generally do not play a central role in the treatment of pain of the severity commonly encountered in cancer patients. They do, however, provide an important and often underutilized adjunctive role that should not be neglected in the patient who is falling just short of adequate pain control (Moertel 1980).

Aspirin, because of its homely appearance, is often overlooked as an effective means of augmenting narcotics. However, like any of the nonnarcotic analgesics, the simple addition of a few aspirin tablets can significantly boost the effect of a narcotic. Aspirin has the disadvantage of causing stomach irritation and can interfere with blood-clotting mechanisms, which make its use hazardous in patients with certain malignancies or ulcer disease. Through gradual losses of small amounts of blood from the stomach, long-term aspirin use can result in anemia; this can be clinically confusing in a patient with a malignancy who may then need to have a variety of other reasons for anemia explored. Its use is contraindicated in patients taking methotrexate since it substantially increases the toxicity of that drug (Moertel 1980).

Acetaminophen (Tylenol), another analgesic augmenter, has fewer gastrointestinal and hematologic adverse effects than aspirin. At high doses, it can be toxic to the liver and kidney. It is important, therefore, that patients tell their physician if they are supplementing their analgesic regimen with over-the-counter drugs such as aspirin or acetaminophen. All medications are potentially involved in drug interactions and create toxic side effects under some circumstances.

Recently, the large class of nonsteroidal anti-inflammatory agents has received recognition for its analgesic potential. This class includes such drugs as ibuprofen (Motrin), naproxen (Naprosyn), and zomepirac (Zomax) (Lewis 1981). This group of drugs can also cause some gastric irritation. Zomepirac, taken orally, appeared to have some potential for a special role since it was found to provide analgesia equivalent to about 10 mg of intramuscular morphine (Forrest 1980; Wallenstein et al. 1980), to have an onset of action in about 30 minutes and a duration of analgesic activity of at least four hours at a time (Cooper 1980; Forrest 1980; Wallenstein et al. 1980), and not to show evidence of physical tolerance or withdrawal symptoms even when used for a period of one year (O'Brien and Minn 1980). However, due to reports of anaphylaxis this drug has been removed from the market. One of the major drawbacks to drugs of this category is their high cost. The nonsteroidal anti-flammatory agents probably work through inhibition of the biosynthesis of prostaglandins and other substances that play a role in inflammation and pain sensitization in the body outside the central nervous system (CNS). They are, therefore, often referred to as "peripheral" agents as opposed to the opioids (narcotics), which work directly within the "central" nervous system. Drugs such as phenylbutazone (Butazolidin), indomethacin (Indocin), and mefenamic acid (Ponstel) also have anti-inflammatory and analgesic activity. Still, their effectiveness in general does not exceed that of aspirin or acetaminophen and their adverse effects and cost are much greater.

Narcotic (Opiate) Analgesics

Generally, all narcotics have similar effects; therefore, as a prescribing principle it is better to use one to its full advantage rather than to switch from one to another in search of some "special" response. It is not uncommon to see pain patients who have been on four or five different narcotics at different doses over several weeks without achieving adequate pain relief. Unfortunately, when the medication record is carefully examined, it often is found that at no time over the two weeks did the patient receive any one of the drugs in a sufficiently high dose.

DETERMINING DOSE.   Within the class of narcotic analgesics, any particular agent is not more or less powerful than any others since any two narcotics can be made to demonstrate equivalent potency by dose alterations. Therefore, it is not the drug itself that is the key variable in analgesia, but the dose, schedule, and route of administration of the drug. Route is important since, as table 6.1

TABLE 6.1
Narcotic Equivalencies

	I.M. Dose (p.o. roughly x 2)	Duration (hours)
Methadone	10	4–6†
Morphine	10	4–5
Hydromorphone (Dilaudid)	1.5	4–5
Oxycodone* (Percodan)	10–15	4–5
Levorphanol (Levo-dromoran)	2–3	4–5
Meperidine (Demerol)	80–100	2–4
Heroin	3	3–4
Codeine		4–6
Pentazocine	60	

*Do not forget presence of other components in Percodan, as large doses of aspirin can result in bleeding complications and large doses of phenacetin may lead to renal papillary necrosis.
†When taken regularly, the analgesic half-life of oral methadone often can be eight hours.
Source: Goldberg, R.J.: *Strategies in psychiatry for the primary physician.* Darien, Conn.: Patient Care Publications, 1980. Used with permission of the Publisher.

demonstrates, drugs taken orally are generally much less potent than drugs given as a "shot," that is, intramuscularly (I.M.). This is important to appreciate since one typical pain problem arises when the physician attempts to switch the patient off I.M. injections and onto oral medication. The transition to taking medication p.o. (by mouth) is important for a variety of reasons, not the least of which is that the patient on oral medication has greater degrees of freedom and autonomy and becomes less dependent on health providers. However, problems in making this switch often arise because of a lack of appreciation for the significant drop in potency that occurs when the same drug is taken by mouth rather than injection. Continuous subcutaneous infusion of morphine has also been used for controlling pain of terminal malignancy (Campbell et al. 1983).

Morphine represents the standard against which narcotics are classically compared. There appears to be no ceiling to the analgesic effect of morphine and progressively higher doses can be used to arrive at complete analgesia. Doses are, however, limited by adverse effects, such as respiratory depression, nausea, and sedation. Though not a factor in limiting dose, constipation accompanies all narcotics and frequently requires coprescribing of a stool softener and some attention to proper diet. While all the narcotics are of equal efficacy if given at equivalent dosages, the effective analgesic duration of narcotics are different and important to remember. Many patients receiving meperidine (Demerol) injections, for example, will begin to complain of pain about 3½ hours after the last injection. Rather than representing a preoccupation with medication, such requests are simply accurate reporting on the drug's rate of metabolism, since its duration of effective action (sometimes referred to as its half-life) is around three hours. (Half-life is the time it takes for half of the amount of drug present to be metabolized.) Therefore, the common practice of ordering meperidine on an every-four-hour (q.4h.) basis is irrational. Knowing the therapeutic duration of the drug being used is crucial in determining how widely to space doses. Generally speaking, longer acting drugs have an advantage of freeing the patient from the necessity of organizing life around medication. For this reason, many physicians advocate the use of methadone (Morgan and Penovich 1977). Methadone has several distinct advantages over the other narcotics generally available. First of all, unlike morphine it has a reasonably good oral potency. Second, its duration of effect is about four hours (which in itself is not a special advantage over several other agents); however, it appears that with regular use the effective analgesic duration of methadone lengthens out so that patients often report good pain control on dose schedules of every six or eight hours. This phenomenon, though not clearly explained, can be of inestimable value to a patient who for the first time is freed from drug taking for major portions of the day, and who begins to have longer stretches of uninterrupted sleep. Generally, methadone's advantages are underappreciated and underutilized. The longer duration, however, can be a disadvantage, especially in older patients for whom the prolonged duration of action can lead to cumulative toxic effects.

Different patients require different doses. There is no magic number of milligrams that can be predicted to work for any particular patient in any specific situation. For example, morphine is often thought of as being used in 10 mg doses and meperidine (Demerol) in 50- or 75-mg doses. However, there is actually nothing standard about these numbers. In determining dose, the most important factor to consider is the effect on the patient. While some patients may do fine on 75 mg of meperidine, another may require 125 mg or 175 mg under circumstances that appear to be similar. There is no substitute for ongoing communication between the patient and the physician.

There is some debate as to whether it is preferable to prescribe medication on a regular schedule or to encourage the patient to take it "as needed" (p.r.n.). Generally, severe pain is better treated on a schedule, for several reasons. When provided "as needed," the patient often experiences the reemergence of pain before taking the next dose of medication, which causes unnecessary suffering. This approach may be irrational because the dose required to abolish pain is larger then the dose required to prevent its reemergence (Reuler et al. 1980; Shimm et al. 1979). At times, especially if other people are responsible for providing the medication when requested, there will be unavoidable delays, leading again to unnecessary suffering or the development of a conditioned anxiety. That is, when medication is given intermittently on an "as needed" basis, the patient is exposed to a powerful reinforcement schedule. Such scheduling in essence "teaches" the patient to be anxious and to complain to obtain medication. It also places the patient in an excessively dependent position. Unfortunately, when such a patient begins to "push the call button" or hang around the nurses' station a half hour before medication is due, he/she becomes stigmatized as someone preoccupied with drugs. As an alternative, medication may be prescribed by a method by which the patient is offered medication on a regular basis, but may refuse it if desired. This method, sometimes referred to as "reverse p.r.n.," ensures that the medication is available, but also helps the patient maintain some autonomy over titrating the dose.

PHYSICAL TOLERANCE.   The development of physical tolerance is a common problem that must be recognized. As the CNS "gets used to" the presence of narcotics, the intensity and duration of drug action lessen. The patient who continues to use narcotics regularly thus will need a higher dose at a briefer interval to get the same results. Unfortunately, this straightforward pharmacologic fact is often overlooked and instead the long-term patient's requests for more medication are often interpreted as evidence of some psychological problem, perhaps the early signs of the dreaded "addiction." The exact time schedule for the development of tolerance varies and cannot be routinely predicted. Increments in doses to make up for effects of tolerance may be needed as soon as several weeks; however, it is not uncommon for patients to be able to go much longer on a stable dose and time schedule. It should always be kept in mind that the need for increasing analgesia may also represent an advance in the underlying disease rather than the emergence of a tolerance effect.

UNRECOGNIZED WITHDRAWAL SYMPTOMS.   Patients who are rapidly switched from high to low doses of narcotics often have some withdrawal symptoms superimposed on the underlying pain symptoms. For this reason, Table 6.2 is included to show the symptoms of narcotic withdrawal and the different time frames for thier appearance. Patients abruptly switched from narcotics to nonnarcotics, or those who through some oversight are given a drug with narcotic antagonist properties, such as pentazocine (Talwin), along with a pure narcotic will have withdrawal symptoms that often are not clearly identified. For this reason, pentazocine (Talwin) should never be given to a patient who is taking other narcotics. The victim of unsuspected drug withdrawal is aware of feeling worse, is often more irritable and physically uncomfortable, and may be mislabeled as a ''complaining'' patient rather than as a patient suffering from drug withdrawal. At other times, the symptoms of withdrawal, such as increased anxiety and pulse rate, will be mistakenly ascribed to an increase in pain.

> Ms. Lilly V. is a 34-year-old, married mother of three children, who has been in the hospital for two weeks for diagnosis and management of pain in her vertebrae and ribs, assumed to represent metastases from an underlying breast cancer. Her bone scans were positive in a number of areas matching her complaints, and she was expected to respond well to radiotherapy. However, several weeks later her pain complaints continued unabated and, to everyone's consternation, actually increased. After she pulled out her intravenous line in an angry gesture, a psychiatric consultant was called to help with her ''childish whining and complaining.'' Upon reviewing her medication orders, the consultant found that her narcotic doses had been on a roller coaster. Because several physicians, nurses, and residents all had different views of how much pain she ''really'' had, her orders reflected ambivalence and a lack of coordination in her treatment plan. For several days she had received the equivalent of 80 mg of morphine, given as 50 mg of meperidine (Demerol) every eight hours, 2 mg of hydromorphone (Dilaudid) as needed every three to four hours, and 5 mg of methadone every four hours. As a reaction to this perceived excess, one attending covering her case abruptly

TABLE 6.2
Abstinence Signs in Narcotic Use

Abstinence Grade	Signs	Morphine	Heroin	Meperidine	Methadone	Codeine	Dihydromorphinone
0	Drug craving Anxiety	6	8	2–3	24	8	2–3
1	Yawning Lacrimation Rhinorrhea Diaphoresis	14	12–18	4–6	36	24	4–6
2	Increase in above Mydriasis Hot-cold flashes Aching bones and muscles Anorexia Muscle twitches Piloerection	16		8–12	48	48	8–12

(Continued on next page)

151

TABLE 6.2
(Continued)

Abstinence Grade	Signs	Morphine	Heroin	Meperidine	Methadone	Codeine	Dihydromorphinone
3	Increase in above Insomnia Increase in blood pressure Increase in temperature Increase in respiratory rate Increase in pulse Restlessness Nausea	24–36	18–24	16	60	—	16
4	Increase in above Fetal position Vomiting Diarrhea Spontaneous ejaculation or orgasm Hemoconcentration	36–48	24–36	—	72	—	16

Source: Goldberg, R.J.: *Strategies in psychiatry for the primary physician.* Darien, Conn.: Patient Care Publications, Inc., 1980. Used with permission of the Publisher.

changed her to oral tablets of acetaminophen (Tylenol) and codeine every four hours—which represented a significant drop in her narcotic use and led predictably to withdrawal symptoms, such as increased anxiety and physical discomfort, on top of her pain. Her "childish" behavior in fact represented the plight of her physical distress associated with severe narcotic withdrawal. Her "personality" problems, as well as her pain, were stabilized by using adequate narcotic doses more consistently, from which she was successfully tapered three weeks later without incident.

Given some education about the pharmacology of narcotics, their risks and benefits, and issues in prescribing, many patients seem quite capable of becoming important collaborators in their own prescribing schedules, using the physician as more of a consultant. Thus, in the classical hospice approach, the patient has medication (often Brompton's solution) always available by the bedside for use whenever he/she feels it is required (Mount et al. 1975). Under such circumstances, there rarely have been reports of any adverse consequences. Such an approach naturally requires physicians and nurses who are comfortable with turning over some of the control normally reserved for the professional; however, the benefit accrued to the patient in terms of the psychological gain can be remarkable. Should patients or physicians increase doses excessively, some of the toxic effects of narcotics, as listed in Table 6.3, may be noted.

Are there, then, any important differences among the narcotics? Generally there are not, except for some variation in *relative*

TABLE 6.3
Signs of Opiate Intoxication

Progressive signs: flusing, itching skin, miosis, drowsiness, decreased respiratory rate, drop in blood pressure and pulse rate, drop in temperature.

Meperidine in high doses (1200 mg/day) may produce muscular twitching, seizures, and signs of toxic psychosis, especially if there is renal impairment. Aside from meperidine, the presence of seizures indicates that some other medical condition is present, such as: mixed addiction (barbiturates), epilepsy, or intracranial pathology.

Also be aware of other medical complications reported in association with narcotic overdoses: pulmonary edema, acute renal failure, myoglobinuria.

potency, time effects, and oral efficacy. Nevertheless, it is undeniable that some patients will do better on one narcotic than some other. Some patients will experience disabling side effects, such as oversedation, or disturbing adverse reactions, such as confusion or agitation, which are not present on an equianalgesic dose of some other narcotic. There has been considerable debate about the use of heroin versus morphine. Heroin has been a widely used narcotic analgesic in England and is included in the original Brompton's formulas as part of hospice care; see "The Brompton Cocktail" (1979).

Brompton's solution.   Brompton's formula is an analgesic recipe prepared from a number of ingredients as an elixer. The combined use of morphine and cocaine to treat pain associated with advanced cancer was first advocated in 1896 (Snow). It was reintroduced 30 years later in Brompton Hospital, from which its name is derived. While there are now some variations in the recipe, it usually consists of heroin (morphine is usually substituted in the United States), alcohol, cocaine, a phenothiazine, chloroform water, and flavoring. This combination touches in some way most of the brain centers associated with pain perception and it is no surprise that it has achieved success and recognition. Some people have contended that heroin provides superior analgesia to other narcotics and has been a victim of discrimination in the United States. However, studies have now revealed no special properties for heroin to support such contention (Melzack et al. 1979; Kiako et al. 1981). Patients thus should not feel deprived if they do not receive heroin. Nor, for that matter, does Brompton's solution provide any unique result that cannot be achieved using other drugs to their full advantage (Melzack et al. 1979).

"Mixed Narcotics."   Some of the drugs considered to be narcotics possess mixed properties, some of which are actually antagonistic to their narcotic effects. Among this class of mixed drugs are pentazocine (Talwin), butorphanol (Stadol), and nalbuphine (Nubain). The presence of some antagonistic properties gives this group certain liabilities and, presumably, certain advantages (Houde 1979). In terms of liabilities, we believe that pentazocine should be avoided altogether because of the high incidence of dysphoric psychological reactions it induces, including feelings of depersonalization and hallucinations. Such psychiatric side effects also occur with butorphanol and are reported least for nalbuphine. Further, if any of these "mixed" drugs is added inadvertently to a narcotic regimen, it can precipitate symptons of narcotic withdrawal (see Table 6.2). Therefore, if a drug from this group is going to be used at all, it must be given early in the course of treatment, before prolonged use of pure narcotics has resulted in the development of physicial dependence. In terms of advantages, this group may produce less nausea and vomiting than other narcotics; have less dependence liability; and tolerance to the analgesic effect may develop more slowly than with the other pure narcotics (especially for nalbuphine) (Vandam 1980). Butorphanol (Stadol, Dorphanol) appears to be about three to five times as potent as morphine in treatment of cancer-associated pain (Heel et al. 1978). The main side effects seem to be sedation and mental confusion. Compared with morphine, there appears to be less respiratory depression with increasing doses (Popio et al. 1978). At this time, however, the role for these "mixed" narcotic agonist-antagonists is uncertain and many clinicians remain unfamiliar with their use.

Drugs that Augment Narcotic Analgesics

Tricyclic antidepressants have received some attention as having analgesic potency in their own right as well as serving to augment other analgesics (Carasso et al. 1979; Lee and Spencer. 1977; Tofanetti et al. 1977). Naturally, symptoms of depression may lead to an exaggerated perception of persistent pain and pain may lead to depressive symptoms. It is somewhat difficult to sort out whether the usefulness of antidepressants in the management of a particular patient is due to a reduction of depressive symptoms or whether, in addition, there has been some analgesic effect. It appears that both actions are likely when antidepressants are used over a period of several weeks. The processing of pain impulses by the CNS involves a number of neurotransmitters, including serotonin. It has been demonstrated in animals that pain sensitivity is lowered by depleting them of this substance. That is, if depleted of serotonin, less severe pain stimuli will produce more noxious responses. This process can be reversed by repleting the serotonin. Interestingly, since the same substance has been implicated in the etiology of some forms of depression, there is a rationale for the addition of antidepressants to a pain regimen with the possibility of achieving three effects at once: analgesics will be augmented, underlying depressive symptoms may be alleviated, and, if given at bedtime, the antidepressant may serve as a hypnotic, thus lessening the need for other sleeping medication. Antidepressants typically used for these purposes include amitriptyline (Elavil), doxepin (Sinequan, Adapin), and maprotiline (Ludiomil). Desyrel (Trazadone), may have some advantages as it produces changes in serotonin systems but has virtually no anticholinergic activity, thereby eliminating some of the tricyclic side effects. (See chapter 4 for further discussion of the use of antidepressants in cancer patients.)

Amphetamines and Cocaine

It has been demonstrated that amphetamines increase the effectiveness of narcotic analgesics (Forrest et al. 1977). This effect does not seem to occur simply on the basis of an energy boost, but rather from some alteration in neurotransmitter function related to pain perception. The use of amphetamine, therefore, may have an important "two-for-one" effect in selected patients. Not only may it augment analgesia, but it can decrease the debilitating effects of somnolence that so often accompany high doses of narcotics. Advanced cancer patients on high doses of morphine need not be somnolent all day and unable to interact with other people or activities. The addition of, for example, 10 mg of dextroamphetamine (Dexedrine) or methylphenidate (Ritalin) in the morning can have a significant alerting effect that may last through much of the day. Some of the side effects of the amphetamine, however, can be problematic. Specifically, tolerance to its effects often occurs within a few weeks, leading to the need for higher doses. If dosage gets too high, for example, over 40 mg, there is some risk of psychiatric side effects, including paranoia or hallucinations. More commonly, amphetamines are known to suppress appetite and interfere with sleep, especially if the dose is taken later than noontime.

Cocaine is the most potent euphoriant known. Because of its stimulant and alerting properties, it has been included as part of the classic recipe in Brompton's solution. There has been a long-standing debate as to whether the inclusion of cocaine was of any significance, since pharmacologists considered oral cocaine to be ineffective, except for the small amount absorbed through the oral mucosa. However, the effectiveness of oral cocaine is now well documented (Wilkinson et al. 1980). Its ability to augment analgesia in a way analogous to amphetamine is theoretically present since there are similarities in their effects on neurotransmitters. The use of psychoactive euphoriants or hallucinogens (such as LSD) as adjuncts for severely ill patients is a relatively unexplored area currently embroiled in controversy.

Hydroxyzine (Vistaril) is an antihistamine commonly used to enhance narcotic analgesics. It has been demonstrated to have some analgesic effect of its own (100 mg of hydroxyzine equal approximately 8 mg of morphine (Bellville et al. 1979). Perhaps this effect accounts for its reputation as an augmenter of narcotic analgesia. Sedation is the main side effect.

Neuroleptics also appear to enhance narcotic analgesics independently of their sedative properties (Moore et al. 1963). Haloperidol (Haldol) is actually a derivative of meperidine (Demerol) and has been established to potentiate morphine analgesics both acutely and chronically (Head et al. 1979). Neuroleptics may be an appropriate choice as an element of pain management when the patient has significant agitation and confusion from an organic mental disorder (see chapter 4) concomitantly with a pain syndrome.

While the adjunctive use of antidepressants or stimulants can play an important role in patient care (Bouckoms 1981), they should not be considered substitutes for the primary consideration in the treatment of pain—that is, the use of adequate doses of analgesics and appropriate attention to the psychosocial factors that influence pain experiences.

Other Somatic Approaches to Pain Relief

While the presence of severe pain naturally leads people to consider narcotic analgesics as the remedy, a number of other nonmedication approaches should be considered. Ice massage is an overlooked, relatively simple means of dealing with local pain. Basically, a painful area is rubbed with ice for approximately ten to 15 minutes to produce an anesthetic effect. Patients are often able to achieve significant pain relief, which can last for hours.

When used at bedtime, the results allow sleep to occur without requiring drug inducement. Only previous frostbite to the area or special sensitivity to cold limits it use.

Another recent development is transcutaneous nerve stimulation (TCNS). This method utilizes small electrodes attached to the skin in the painful region and stimulated by a low-intensity current supplied by a portable battery unit. It has virtually no side effects and appears to work best in myofacial syndromes, peripheral nerve injuries, and phantom limb and stump pain (Melzack 1975). While obtaining pain relief, the patient will feel only a mild tingling or sensation in the area of the electrodes. This form of analgesia is, unfortunately, unsatisfactory for those forms of pain that do not appear to have a peripheral cause.

Anxiety augments pain perception. Therefore, any means of regulating anxiety may allow patients to get relief from lower doses of narcotics (Turk and Rennert 1981). There are a number of self-regulating techniques (Goldberg 1982) that can be learned in a brief period of time by most people. It is frustrating when the physician tells the patient simply to "relax," since many people do not know how. Unfortunately, most physicians are not prepared by a classical medical education to teach relaxation methods. But fortunately, there is an increasing number of self-teaching aids available in this area, as well as oncology programs that increasingly offer the services of someone to assist patients in learning self-regulatory methods of anxiety reduction such as muscle relaxation, muscle biofeedback, and meditation.

Psychosocial Components of Pain Management

Patient–Hospital Staff Dysfunction

It is assumed that most patients will achieve pain control given adequate and appropriate amounts of analgesia. However, pain remains a problem for many people because of a series of predictable and preventable psychological and interpersonal events (Goldberg 1980). What happens when a patient remains in pain despite the routine approach used by the physician? And how can a nurse or social worker involved with the patient assist in such cases? The response to inadequately treated pain depends, of course, on the personality of the patient (Goldberg 1983). Those people who are not inclined to speak out and who are somewhat intimidated by authority may withdraw and keep their reactions hidden. Such silent sufferers are rarely given a second thought by health care providers who, in a world of cascading demands, tend to overlook quiet patients in favor of applying oil to the squeaky wheels. Quiet patients are generally considered good patients. Occasionally, some astute person will identify social withdrawal as a sign of possible depression and prompt psychiatric attention. In such cases, the problem is the patient's sense of helplessness rather than depression (also see chapter 3 for a discussion of medical disorders that lead to behavioral symptoms such as social withdrawal). Depressive symptoms emerge in the context of prolonged pain *via* a learned helplessness model in which the patient's experience is that, "Nothing I do seems to matter anyway, so why try?"

More assertive individuals may respond to inadequate pain relief by complaining loudly and regularly. While assertiveness may be adaptive to survival on one level, it carries some risks if it becomes viewed by providers as extreme. The patient at times treads a thin line between complaining so as to alert people that something is not working, and complaining so much that people stop listening. Patients feel it is important to have doctors and nurses like them. When one seems to be in a position of dependence on the good will of caretakers, it takes some courage to test the staff's maturity by complaints, which imply criticism. Complaining, of course, may lead to a positive response, or to a worsening of the problem (Figure 6.1). Patients viewed as excessive complainers often begin to lose credibility. Remarks overheard at the nurse's station might include, "That patient doesn't seem to be in so much pain, so why should she be complaining so much? She can't still be in all that much pain after the amount of medication she has received." Once a patient's credibility is questioned by the staff, the general tenor of treatment shifts in subtle but significant ways. Everything the patient says begins to be examined more carefully and the patient becomes a potential "problem." The risk of creating a credibility gap is most significant for the patient who is characteristically voluble, demonstrative, or a bit histrionic. Certain cultural groups are socioculturally programmed to display emotions in ways that are difficult for the medical care system to manage (Fabrega and Tyma 1976; Streltzer and Wade 1981), inasmuch as scientific medicine functions most efficiently with well-controlled, verbal, articulate, cooperative patients, whose

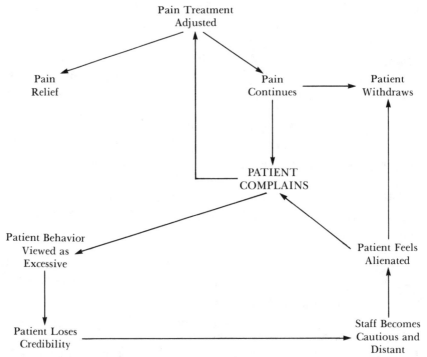

FIGURE 6.1   Systems Dysfunction in Pain Management

feelings are generally under control or denied. Overt displays of emotion are difficult for a medical system since the survival of the system depends on the elimination of the excessive charges of emotion that constantly threaten to overwhelm the participants. Mechanisms to distance and depersonalize death and suffering are built into the framework of medical care. Therefore, the histrionic patient is at higher risk for creating a gap between patient and staff.

Distancing by the staff has its own adverse consequences. Patients whose very lives seem dependent on the interaction with a few caretakers become extremely sensitive to the nuances within the caretaking relationship. Any sense of increased distance or widening of the communication gap can create a sense of alienation.

Feelings of isolation are ever present in our health care system. It is unfortunate that, because of a significant and growing shortage of hospital nurses in the United States, there are simply not enough nurses on each shift to be able to get all the work done in such a way that the individual needs of the patients are always met on time. The more difficult patients generally seem to be affected most by getting less of what is available when there is less to go around. It is understandable for nurses to try to get some gratification out of their difficult work by spending more time with those patients who are most likely to return something positive. Pain patients who are viewed as problem patients may accurately perceive the negative staff attitude toward them, though that sense often becomes exaggerated for those who dependency needs lead to excessive fears of abandonment. The patient's sense of abandonment ("no one listens to me anymore") leads to an increased fearfulness that can lead to further compensatory, often maladaptive, behaviors, such as talking about wanting to leave the hospital or to drop out of treatment. Such desperate maneuvers, which can be understood as induced by a dysfunction in the treatment system, add to staff discomfort even more and augment the problem. (See Figure 6.1.)

The Misuse of Placebo

A placebo is an inert substance (usually an injection of saline solution) or a "sugar pill" given to a patient who is suspected of not having "real" pain. Unfortunately, there remains significant misunderstanding about placebos within some sectors of the medical and nursing professions. The patient whose complains of pain are viewed as exaggerated is, in some units, a likely candidate for a placebo.

Placebos are widely used in the hospital setting for a variety of reasons (Goldberg et al. 1979), including treatment of pain, when "routine" treatment fails, and when the basis for pain is thought to be largely "emotional." Placebo use is often rationalized as a means of helping patients avoid other more "dangerous" treatments and as a diagnostic tool that can help the staff decide whether the pain is "real."

> Timothy R. is a 22-year-old unemployed man who required amputation of his left leg for osteogenic sarcoma. Following the surgical procedure, the patient complained about unrelieved pain both at the sites of surgery and in the "phantom limb." In his follow-up treatment, he received doses of narcotics that most likely were too low and too infrequent to result in

good pain control. The typical cycle described in the previous section emerged. As the patient's complaints became more scathing and "unreasonable," he was transformed in the eyes of the staff from an "unfortunate victim" into an "unreliable" and "immature" person interested in "getting drugs." He was felt to be crying out in excess of the amount of pain that was "really there."

Such a situation is an ideal breeding ground for the use of placebo. Inevitably, someone suggests that the patient be given an injection of saltwater instead of a narcotic to "see what happens." It is important to know that a significant portion of the population (about 30 to 40%) are placebo "responders." That is, many people will get some transient relief of virtually any symptom following a placebo. Pain associated with documented advanced disease, such as carcinoma in the pancreas, kidney stones, or severe trauma, often can be successfully and reliably relieved by placebo. But such relief is only transient, and the more the placebo is used, the less relief it provides. Since both "real" and "imagined" pain will respond transiently to placebo, *placebo has no value whatsoever as a diagnostic tool*. Placebo analgesia actually may take place because of induction of endorphin activity and may therefore have a physiologic, not totally a psychological, basis (Levine et al. 1978). Nevertheless, in Timothy's case, when the saline injection resulted in some temporary relief of pain, the staff accepted this as confirmation of their suspicions that his complaints were not warranted by any underlying medical/surgical problem. As a result, Timothy's analgesic regimen was lowered further. When his behavior became more irrational, a psychiatric consultant was called. The misinterpretation of the response placebo was clarified, and the vicious cycle of patient–staff interaction was broken by the consultant taking responsibility for increasing the narcotics. Finally, relieved of pain, Timothy was no longer a "problem" patient.

Placebo use emerges from both a combination of misunderstanding of what it can accomplish and some patient–staff conflict. Rather than addressing the underlying issue, placebo use only serves further to alienate patient and staff since it requires "lying" to the patient and therefore creates a further credibility gap. Whenever placebo use is contemplated by the staff, the clinician should ask, "What is happening in this treatment system?" Typical answers include: Inadequate narcotic medication is being used; the personality style of the patient has prompted the staff to become unduly suspicious; and/or the ongoing nature of the patient–staff interaction is caught in conflict. While the patient, of course, will not be told that he/she is being given a placebo, the family or consultant who becomes aware of its use should raise some questions about what is going on.

The Private Meaning of Pain

No symptom is experienced in a psychological vacuum. For most people, a physical symptom brings to mind something that happened to somebody else. Knee pain may remind the person of a newspaper article about a young boy whose leg required amputation for a cancer discovered accidentally as a small painful bump. Midwinter cough and fatigue may be just the flu, or the harbinger of lung cancer, which was diagnosed in a colleague following the same symptoms. Family histories create especially powerful mythologies. Anyone with significant medical or psychiatric illness running in the family knows that reason often falls short of settling the deep-seated uneasiness that destiny holds a common fate for the family. For families with cancer (it has recently been estimated that two out of three American families will have a member experience cancer), seemingly insignificant physical symptoms can portend catastrophe. Fortunately, most people, while healthy, are able to maintain an adaptive denial about such private thoughts.

One factor that commonly interferes with routine pain control is the psychological blurring of one's own experience with someone else's. "I saw what it was like for Aunt Ethel and assume my experience will be at least as bad." Some patients whose pain symptoms are not responsive to conventional approaches may be victims of psychological associations that are powerfully overdetermined by memories, past experiences, or symbolic overtones of the experience. With cases of nonresponsive pain, the clinician should always ask: "Do you know or have you heard of anyone else who had a problem like this. If so, what happened to that person?"

Roberta is a middle-aged woman who was admitted to the hospital for treatment of chronic headache, not responsive to high doses of Fiorinal. The headache had been severe and virtually constant for about a week and continued in the hospital despite relatively high dose narcotics. A computerized axial tomographic (CAT) scan and spinal tap were negative and a psychiatric consultant was called. In the very first interview, the consultant found out what everyone else knew, that the patient's mother died of a subarachnoid hemorrhage (bleeding within the brain), but went a step further to find out the details of the death. The patient, in an increasingly emotional outpouring, described how her mother literally had died in her arms. They had been sitting in the living room together, listening to the radio, when her mother suddenly grabbed her head, vomited, and slumped over into the patient's lap, dying moments later. The mother had complained of a bad headache all that day. Though all this had happened more than ten years before, this was the first time Roberta had ever discussed it in any detail and allowed herself any emotional release. By the end of the interview, her headache was gone and she was soon discharged from the hospital.

While this case is stunningly dramatic, it represents a not uncommon problem of how unresolved grief becomes intermingled with pain experiences and how the exploration of important personal losses can be therapeutic for the patient in pain. Exaggerated fantasies of damage following surgery can also augment the psychological experience of pain. Some people develop distorted and overly destructive images of what has gone on inside their bodies as a result of cancer or its treatment. It is not unusual for the image of disfigurement or internal destruction powerfully to influence pain perception. Reassurance about the healing process can lay such excessive anxiety to rest.

Further Considerations

Pain is a private experience created by dimensions that include the biologic, psychological, and social. The majority of pain problems can be adequately managed by the knowledgeable application of standard pharmacologic approaches. Many pain patients are wrongly assumed to be "immature" or a "complaining type" when actually their difficult behavior is a direct outcome of inadequate treatment and inappropriate responses of nurses and physicians. The magnified fear of addiction by pain patients and professionals is one of the greatest obstacles to pain management.

It is difficult to accept as definitive a medical evaluation of pain that turns up empty-handed. When should one accept that the symptom has been fully evaluated? There are some pain consultants who have the attitude that all pain is the result of some identifiable medical disorder and leave no stone unturned. For example, a significant number of lung cancer patients have back pain secondary to metastatic involvement of the vertebral column, a process that can usually be diagnosed by a bone scan of that area. However, it has recently been pointed out that in a significant number of patients with such pain the scan will appear normal despite the fact that metastatic involvement will later prove to be present (Covelli et al. 1980). Good doctors are aware that there are definite limitations in diagnostic tests. Despite a negative bone scan, many lung cancer patients with back pain do quite well when empirically given irradiation to the painful areas of the back. While some exhaustive searches for the source of unexplained pain do uncover some overlooked medical problem, many of them only serve to provide the patient with added expense, discomfort, and false hopes.

Role of the Psychosocial Consultant

Non-responsive pain is an appropriate indication for involvement of a psychiatric consultant. The ensuing evaluation should address possible biological, psychological, and social dimensions of the pain as discussed in this chapter. The evaluation is best initiated by a history of the symptom which gathers information on two levels—the "objective" data, such as time of onset, treatments, providers, complications, etc.; and the "subjective" experiences associated with each event, including elicitation of fears, or disappointments associated with treatment.

The psychosocial consultant must also have some awareness of the medical issues involved in diagnosis to participate in a meaningful way. If not a physician, it is important that the consultant function as a member of a multidisciplinary team in which this dimension of care can be considered by a psychiatrist who is knowledgeable in the area. However, understanding the systems context of pain treatment goes beyond the pharmacology alone. Beyond the issue of the biomedical dimension, the consultant should consider whether the patient's personality is a problem for the providers or whether there is an issue between the physicians and/or the nursing staff and patient that is interfering with rational care.

In addition to the cycle of events reviewed in the previous sections, which leads to a sense of alienation for the patient, having multiple providers commonly fosters problems in pain management. Because the complexity of modern technology often brings multiple specialties to bear on the treatment of a single patient, there may be confusion from time to time about who is in charge and whose orders take precedence. As difficult as it is to work out a rational pain regime with one patient and one doctor, good care becomes virtually unworkable with many doctors and housestaff. One of the most common interventions necessary in the management of "unresponsive" pain patients is the identification of one person to be in charge of medication orders.

The patient, family, and consultants should not collude by standing by confused when pain seems excessive. Knowledge of medication can help people become more effective advocates for their own care. Finally, when there seem to be tensions between the patient and staff, a psychiatric consultation (see chapter 9) is often successful in disrupting the interpersonal distortions that can emerge in the context of the anguish and frustrations of pain.

References

ANGELL, M.: The quality of mercy. *N. Engl. J. Med.* 306 (1982): 98–99.

BELLVILLE, J. W., DOREY, F., CAPPARELL, D., KNOX, V., AND BAUER, R.: Analgesic effects of hydroxyzine compared to morphine in man. *J. Clin. Pharmacol.* 19 (1979): 5–6.

BOUCKOMS, A. J.: Analgesic adjuvants: The role of psychotropics, anticonvulsants, and prostaglandin inhibitors. *Drug Ther. (Hosp.)*(1981): 41–48.

The Brompton cocktail. *Lancet* (1979): 1220–1221.

CAMPBELL, C. F., MASON, J. B., AND WEILER J. M.: Continuous subcutaneous infusion of morphine for the pain of terminal malignancy. *Ann. Intern. Med.* 98 (1983): 51–52.

CARASSO, R. L., YEHUDA, S., AND STREIFLER, M.: Clomipramine and amitriptyline in the treatment of severe pain. *Int. J. Neurosci.* 9 (1979): 191–194.

COOPER, S. A.: Efficacy of zomepirac in oral surgical pain. *J. Clin. Pharmacol.* 20 (1980): 230–242.

COVELLI, H. D., ZALOZNIK, A. J., AND SHEKITKA, K. M.: Evaluation of bone pain in carcinoma of the lung. *JAMA* 244 (1980): 2625–2627.

FABREGA, H., AND TYMA, S.: Language and cultural influences in the description of pain. *Br. J. Med. Psychol.* 49 (1976): 349–371.

FORREST, W. H., JR.: Orally administered zomepirac and parentally administered morphine: Comparison for the treatment of postoperative pain. *JAMA* 244 (1980): 2298–2302.

FORREST, W. H., ET AL.: Dextroamphetamine with morphine for the treatment of postoperative pain. *N. Engl. J. Med.* 296 (1977): 712.

GOLDBERG, R. J.: Anxiety reduction by self-regulation: Theory, practice, and evaluation. *Ann. Intern. Med.* 96 (1982): 483–487.

_____: Pain. In *Strategies in psychiatry for the primary physician.* Darien, Conn.: Patient Care Publications, 1980, chap. 5.

_____: Personality disorders. In H. Leigh (Ed.), *Psychiatry in primary care medicine.* Menlo Park: Addison-Wesley, 1983.

GOLDBERG, R. J., LEIGH, H., AND QUINLAN, D.: The current status of placebo in hospital practice. *Gen. Hosp. Psychiatry* (1979): 196–201.

HEAD, M., ET AL.: Enhancement of morphine analgesia after acute and chronic haloperidol. *Life Sci.* 24 (1979): 2037–2044.

HEEL, R. C., BROGDEN, R. N., SPEIGHT, T. M., AND AVERY, G. S.: Butorphanol: A review of its pharmacological properties and therapeutic efficacy. *Drugs* 16 (1978): 473–505.

HOUDE, R. W.: Analgesic effectiveness of the narcotic agonist-antagonists. *Br. J. Clin. Pharmacol.* 7 (1979): 297S–308S.

KAIKO, R. F., ROGERS, A. G., WALLENSTEIN, S. L., ET AL.: Analgesic and mood effects of heroin and morphine in cancer patients with postoperative pain. *N. Engl. J. Med.* 304 (1981): 1501–1505.

LEE, R., AND SPENCER, P. S. J.: Antidepressants and pain. *J. Intern. Med. Res.* 5 (1977), suppl. 1,: 146–156, 1977.

LEVINE, J. D., GORDON, N. C., AND FIELDS, H. L.: The mechanism of placebo analgesia. *Lancet* (1978): 654–657.

LEWIS, J. R.: Zomepirac sodium. A new nonaddicting analgesic. *JAMA* 246 (1981), 4: 377–379.

MARKS, R. M., AND SACHAR, E. J.: Undertreatment of medical inpatients with narcotic analgesics. *Ann. Intern. Med.* 78 (1973): 173–181.

MCKEGNEY, F. P., BAILEY, L. R., AND YATES, J. W.: Prediction and management of pain in patients with advanced cancer. *Gen. Hosp. Psychiatry* 3 (1981): 95–101.

MELZACK, R., MOUNT, B. M., AND GORDON, J. M.: The brompton mixture versus morphine solution given orally: Effects of pain. *Can. Med. Assoc. J.* 120 (1979): 435–438.

MELZACK, R.: Prolonged relief of pain by brief intense transcutaneous somatic stimulation. *Pain* 1 (1975): 357.

MERSKEY, H., AND SPEAR, F. G.: The concept of pain. *J. Psychosom. Res.* 7: 59–67.

MILLER, R. R., AND JICK, H.: Clinical effects of meperidine in hospitalized medical patients. *J. Clin. Pharmacol.* 18 (1978): 180–189.

MOERTEL, C. G.: Treatment of cancer pain with orally administered medications. *JAMA* 244 (1980), 21: 2448–2450.

MOORE, J., ET AL.: Alterations in response to somatic pain: Pain associated with anaesthesia: VII. The effects of non-phenothiazine derivatives. *Br. J. Anaesth.* 33 (1963): 422–430.

MORGAN, J. P., AND PENOVICH, P.: Methadone: Still an analgesic. *Drug. Ther. (Hosp.)* (1977): 18–23.

MOUNT, B. M., ET AL.: Use of brompton mixture in treating the chronic pain of malignant disease. *Can. Med. Assoc. J.* 1 (1975): 10–18.

O'BRIEN, C. P., AND MINN, F. L.: Evaluation for withdrawal symptoms following chronic zomepirac administration. *J. Clin. Pharmacol.* 20 (1980): 397–400.

POPIO, K. A., JACKSON, D. H., ROSS, A. M., SCHREINER, B. F., AND YU, P. N.: Hemodynamic and respiratory effects of morphine and butorphanol. *Clin. Pharmacol. Ther.* 23: 281–287, 1978.

PORTER, J., AND JICK, H.: Addiction rare in patients treated with narcotics. *N. Engl. J. Med.* 302 (1980): 123.

REULER, J. B., GIRARD, D. E., AND NARDONE, D. A.: The chronic pain syndrome: Misconceptions and management. *Ann. Intern. Med.* 93 (1980): 588–596.

SHIMM, D. S., LOGUE, G. L., MALTBIE, A. A., AND DUGAN, S.: Medical management of chronic cancer pain. *JAMA* 241 (1979): 2408–2412, 1979.

SNOW, H.: Opium and cocaine in the treatment of cancerous disease. *Br. Med. J.* ii (1896): 718.

STRELTZER, J., AND WADE, T. C.: The influence of cultural group on the undertreatment of postoperative pain. *Psychosom. Med.* 43 (1981), 5: 397–403.

TOFANETTI, O., ALBIERO, L., GALATULAS, I., ET AL.: Enhancement of propoxyphene-induced analgesia by Doxepin. *Psychopharmacol* 51 (1977): 213–215.

TURK, D. C., AND RENNERT, K.: Pain and the terminally ill cancer patients: A cognitive-social learning perspective. In H. J., Sobel (Ed.), *Behavior therapy in terminal care, a humanistic approach*. Cambridge, Mass.: Ballinger, 1981.

TWYCROSS, R. G.: Value of cocaine in opiate containing elixirs. *Br. Med. J.* ii (1977): 1348.

VANDAM, L. D.: Drug therapy: Butorphanol. *N. Engl. J. Med.* 302 (1980): 381–384.

WALLENSTEIN, S. L., ROGERS, A., KAIKO, R. F., ET AL.: Relative analgesic potency of oral zomepirac and intramuscular morphine in cancer patients with postoperative pain. *J. Clin. Pharmacol.* 20: 250–258, 1980.

WILKINSON, P., VANDYKE, C., JATLOW, P., ET AL.: Intranasal and oral cocaine kinetics. *Clin. Pharmacol. Ther.* 27 (1980): 386–394.

PART III

Problems for Caregivers and Treatment Programs

CHAPTER 7

Issues for Caregivers

WORKING WITH CANCER PATIENTS often creates special stresses as well as the opportunity for extraordinary personal and professional gratification. Caregivers face the challenge of maintaining some distance from patients while meeting the need for the clinical and personal involvement so crucial to having some therapeutic impact on patients. Among the ways in which organized medical care reduces the emotionally traumatic aspects of contact is the creation of treatment protocols and routinization of tasks (Parsons 1951) that remove the personal element and replace it with social structures. The concern of every caregiver therefore must be to avoid excessively impersonal treatment while at the same time finding a way to metabolize the intense experiences they encounter. One provider's comments reflect an awareness of the task that confronts a sensitive caregiver in the oncology setting:

> I think there is at times almost a slavish adherence to programs of treatment. The people doing that are people who I think hide behind those treatments. I think they are good people, but I think they hide behind them in a way that tells me that the burdens that we have to face caring for oncology patients

are really, really great burdens, burdens that we better prepare ourselves for.

There is no generalizable recipe to assist staff development in this area. Every oncology caregiver possesses a unique blend of personality assets and insecurities. This chapter is intended to help caregivers understand and prepare themselves to overcome some of the stressful forces in this field, which, if neglected, can lead to loss of productivity and satisfaction.

Personal and Social Challenges

Working with cancer patients takes on a mystique as cancer has become a modern metaphor for human confrontation with existential uncertainty. To varying degrees, caregivers may become aware of and be affected by this dramatic dimension of their work. The opportunity for heightened self-awareness can be one of the potentially fulfilling and rewarding aspects of the work; however, such an opportunity does not come without facing some intense professional challenges. Some people may be hesitant to introspect about their work experience or feel that it is unnecessary. Yet being a good clinician requires constant self-examination at some level and reassessment is especially warranted for those who think they may be experiencing "burnout." While no one today seems to be able to escape mention of this term, many do not realize that it applies to them until they review what it means.

Burnout (Freudenberger 1974) refers to the physical, emotional, or behavioral consequences of prolonged exposure to job-related stress. In health care professions, burnout is a primary cause of poor clinical care, professional apathy, cynicism, job turnover, and lowered morale (Maslach 1979). The physical signs and symptoms that have been ascribed to burnout include feelings of exhaustion, of being physically run down; sleep disturbance; depression; and a variety of somatic symptoms including frequent headaches, gastrointestinal disturbances, weight loss, and shortness of breath. Behaviorally, this syndrome is characterized by one or a combination of the following: a tendency to cry easily, a loss of the ability to feel emotionally involved, increased irritability, diminished frustration tolerance, feelings of hopelessness, and, at times, suspiciousness. In addition to increased interpersonal conflicts (Vachon 1979), people experiencing this syndrome are likely to take increased risks that involve poor judgment and are at high risk for involvement with tranquilizers, narcotics, or alcohol. Rigidity of attitude toward co-workers and clinical problems also seems to characterize this syndrome. Stress in some people manifests by creating a rigidity in character, which can lead to inflexibility in behavior and clinical thinking. A lack of flexibility is a special risk in oncology care that occurs at the interface of so many systems and challenges the provider to consider so many uncharted decisions in the medical, ethical, and psychological realms.

Describing what it means for the caregiver to be ''coping'' with the oncology setting is as difficult as it is to define what it means for the patient to be ''coping'' with the disease. Caregivers, like patients, possess a repertoire of coping skills and an inventory of vulnerabilities. Poor coping in caregivers can lead to the maladaptive symptoms of burnout or job termination. However, all unpleasantness encountered in caregivers should not automatically be ascribed to burnout since personal lack of sociability or poor judgment may precede and be independent of the particular setting.

Each staff person makes the best adaptation he or she can manage at the moment. While angry or inflexible behavior of some patients can be understood and addressed in the context of treatment, it is often more difficult to have to live with maladaptive staff behaviors—yet every system is made up of people who may not be ideally suited to their positions.

The purpose of this chapter is not to suggest that everyone be ''made over'' in some ideal form. In fact, it seems to be a mistake to hold up a single clinician model. Suggesting that all caregivers should possess the unique gifts of someone such as Kübler-Ross may even have a negative impact by making some providers feel incompetent. Instead, the purpose of the chapter is to join others (Kolotkin 1981) in helping caregivers become more comfortable with themselves, to put systems issues in perspective, and thereby, it is hoped, to overcome or avoid burnout and to have a vitalizing impact on patient care. This chapter is not meant to be an exhaustive review of every issue facing the caregiver, but rather an opportunity to share some thoughts from other providers. One oncologist, in reflecting on his way of dealing with the field, said:

> Though there are stresses to what I do, the fact is I think by and large it is by choice that I have chosen this path, and I think

that I try to mitigate the stresses by first seeing as best as I can if I can identify in some easily recognizable way what those stresses are and than attempt to at least be up front and say I do or do not know how to handle them.

Identifying the issues is the first step in managing work-related stress.

People may not be prepared to become oncology providers any more than others are prepared to experience cancer. They end up in this field for a variety of reasons. Some have clearly identifiable developmental experience that sheds some light on the choice of working with cancer patients. Such experiences sometimes have to do with an early experience of a cancer death of a friend or relative:

> One of the reasons I'm in oncology was a good friend who died at a young age, age 20. There were a few of us in my neighborhood in Manhattan who grew up together and used to play ball regularly. There were about six or seven of us actually, and one of the group died very suddenly of leukemia. Later on, in studying the process . . . this was at a time when I was in medical school with really not any certainty that I was going into oncology . . . the process of leukemia itself became horrendously, almost mystifyingly, attractive, the process by which the body could go berserk and some component of the body take over in a way that violates and overcomes the rest of the body. It was so horrendous in a way, and yet there was something very exciting about it, something very real in a way that I had just never felt before as I considered other medical specialties.

However, many find themselves in an oncology setting as a result of circumstances such as job availability, willingness to try something new, or the personal impetus to face a challenge:

> I guess I felt that it was going to be difficult for me, and I felt that I really wanted to spend my time for better or worse, and I guess this was part of my ideal of being a physician, working with situations in which the pathology itself is really not in doubt.

Sometimes personality characteristics can be identified that may account for the attraction to the field of oncology:

> I think one factor was coming from my own background, not being particularly popular when young, not being particularly comfortable with peers, perhaps, feeling myself at times al-

most an underdog. That was the word that sort of jumped out of me, connoting to me the attitude of the medical profession towards the oncology patient at that time, being abysmal. Certainly I remember many instances toward the end of my training that I thought of the idea of the underdog in that context, those patients with savage illness.

The initial experience of this specialized area of medicine may seem uneventful. Once in the field, it often takes a while before the person masters the terminology and therapeutics and begins to experience the emotional impact of working in an oncology setting. The initial contact with patients seems not significantly different from many other medical settings; however, for those unaccustomed to working with patients with life-threatening illness, the inexorable progression or chronicity of the disease in the majority of patients soon begins to take its toll. This is not to say that many cancer patients are not being cured; however, the ones who do well may be seen infrequently and with less involvement. Reflecting on the cumulative nature of the response to loss of patients, one nurse said:

> I think that after awhile there is a grieving process that goes on. We feel grief in our own private ways kind of, and I think that after a while you don't get to catch up maybe on your own grieving process. It can drive you crazy.

Symptoms of unresolved grief can be present in a variety of ways. Some may not be aware of this cumulative unresolved grief until, for example, they find themselves crying easily when watching television. Others may find their sleep patterns interrupted or filled with work-related dreams.

> After a few months I began to have dreams about having cancer. One of them was thinking about who would I tell first. It was so vivid. I remember having chemotherapy. I remember having one of those things put on my head with the ice so I wouldn't lose my hair. I felt that there was no getting away from it. It was really something, and identifying with the patients and all.

How people understand and manage their emotional responses to the setting is crucial to their own professional well-being and clinical efficiency. Some, of course, may feel that the emotional toll of working with cancer patients is too great and transfer; however, often because of geographic or personal circumstances, some are unable to change settings so easily. Those who continue to thrive often talk about how their personal development has been enhanced by the experience of working with cancer patients:

> I think that it has made me think about issues that you don't usually face until you're in your late or midlife, things about death. Most people my age, I don't think they think about death, and I've thought about it a lot more.

Such a confrontation can raise spiritual issues or call personal values into question:

> I don't go around thinking that my life may end tomorrow but I guess that it's there in the back of my mind and that maybe it's more important that if I want to do something I do it today. I'm not going to save up all my money for a rainy day or something like that. I think I'm more present oriented than future oriented. I also look at people's reactions to illness and things, I guess, a little bit differently than others would, but I think I was brought up with that in my background.

Few providers in this field can escape the constant reminder of life's transience and the uneasiness that comes from the recognition that even when science does its best, death cannot be overcome. This problem seems most difficult for those with a cure-oriented medical approach as opposed to those who derive satisfaction from a care-oriented approach. The denial of death to which most people cling can be directly eroded by working in the setting. The reaction to such existential insults can be quite varied. Some people discover a greater appreciation for what life offers. Others may find themselves questioning their attitudes toward religion, marriage, medicine, or other institutions, as well as their attitudes toward the balance between self-denial and indulgence. There is also some danger that the work context can be used as a global rationale for any behavior:

> I think it's very tempting to justify a change in values or change in attitudes by what I see, and I think there's a great danger in that, because I think that it is a very special thing that we are exposed to, a very special privilege in a sense that we have in seeing people at their baldest, if you will. I still think that trying to apply the values gained from that in more than a very limited sense to maybe specific instances as they arise is fraught with great danger. In me, I think the tendency would be to, therefore, say that I can justify myself doing things and say-

ing things and feeling things that put down the next guy because he's not experiencing the same kind of stresses; he's not in a sense proceeding through the same kinds of tremendous turmoils and emerging, hopefully, partially scathed but still able to continue. I think there are times when I do feel that I do have a different perspective on life, at least in the sense of trying to live a little more fully, trying to gain a little bit more from each day, and not wait for the right times so called, as one can really never predict what can happen.

There can also be a definite impact on interpersonal relationships and home life. Some providers may begin to feel that they are a special breed, unique inasmuch as an immersion in the drama of life and death creates a perspective they feel others may lack. The concerns and preoccupations of friends may begin to seem insignificant or trifling. Such a divergence of values can create a sense of isolation.

It can be hard to relate to people who are so worried about their hairdos . . . I think our bodies are important, and I exercise, but I mean people who stand there and are so worried about this extra pound or this pimple on their face and things like that. I try not to, but I find it hard to have sympathy for things like that when there are so many more serious things. I think everybody working with cancer patients would feel that way. People get involved with and hung up on things that aren't as important, although to them they're important, I know that, and I think we all do it. I do it too sometimes. Maybe if I weren't a nurse, I would focus on many more trivial things than I do now.

We have been told repeatedly by people in the field that there is a phase when important relationships come into question. After working all day with dying patients, coming home to someone whose concern is that the grass was cut in the wrong direction can seem absurd. There is a phase when providers feel a sense of distance from others who seem to remain sheltered from confronting mortality. This sense of distance can be transient and the provider can reestablish relationships with a greater appreciation for them, with more of an appreciation of the blend of deep emotion and triviality that characterizes most important relationships. It helps not to take oneself too seriously. However, others may find problems in overcoming the sense of incompatability. Those who find themselves having increased interpersonal or marital problems should examine the extent to which the existential strain of their job is partly responsible. Yet work also can be used as an excuse for other sources of incompatability in a relationship and can even provide an excuse for hiding behind or avoiding the relationship. The strain of working in a cancer setting can be the catalyst rather than the direct cause of problems in an interpersonal relationship.

The sense of isolation that can emerge from working with this population can be further augmented by the difficulty in talking about work at home. It can be especially hard to make a transition on a day when you have just experienced the death of two patients with whom you have worked closely for eight months. When you are asked at dinner, "Well, dear, what's new at work?" you feel the answer is not exactly dinnertime conversation, yet the impact of work cannot be denied. Some providers claim "they leave work behind":

> We all have our own problems at home, too, so if you try to bring everything home, it just doesn't work out. I think part of my handling work stress is that I put as much as I can into it while I'm at work and once I'm home, I try to forget about it. There are a few patients I think about, but I don't go home and get very depressed over it. I don't know what that means; I'm not sure. I hope it doesn't mean that I'm hardened and cold, but it's the way I handle it; it's the way I can handle it best.

Others find that their own way to deal with the stress is outside of relationships:

> I sort of value my privacy and I think there are just times where someone will say, "Let's go out," or something, and I'll say, "No, that's all right. I'd rather just stay home today, if that's okay with you." I think that I look things over at those times . . . I'll do things like reading a book or something like that, but I do things . . . or even just clean my house or something, but I think those are the times that I get to catch up on things and sit down and think about things that have happened.

And others find ways to bring the emotions generated at work into their other relationships. A renewed sense of the value of the relationship can also emerge:

> Work has made me think about the nature of my relationships and what kind of support I would want if I had cancer, and how to do that, and how to develop the kind of support in the people that I know that would help me through a traumatic

illness, and it sort of gives me a preparation, and almost to be able to tell somebody, "This is what I need from you now," and knowing who might be able, who has the resources to provide that, and you can look at your relationships in a different way, based on anticipating crisis as you see it in other people and as you know yourself.

Preoccupation with death is an unfortunate way to go through life. At the other extreme, our culture has been criticized for an extreme aversion to death awareness. Yet work in oncology confronts one with death in ways that are palpable and repeated. It can be especially difficult for providers working with a patient of the same sex, age, education, and so on. A typical reaction to such identification was stated by one nurse as follows:

The most difficult patient for me would be a young woman with breast cancer, because I think she's my age now, and I could be that person. Or a young man with seminoma or brain tumor, for example, I think, that could be my husband. That, I think, probably gets me more upset than anything else.

In such situations it is not unusual to find the staff avoiding the patient. It might even be indicated at times to transfer the care of such a patient to another provider who is able to feel more objective. Staff should always be alert to the special strain that can be created for the primary provider, whether nurse or physician, who is caring for a patient with some special self-identification.

Providers may have trouble working with certain patients for reasons other than overidentification because of sex, age, education, or profession. A number of privately held health-related fears and fantasies play a role in the experience of many oncology providers. Providers are not immune from the general public fear that cancer may be contagious. Such concerns are not generally shared, though they certainly seem at times to influence attitudes and behaviors. One social worker shared her concerns in this area saying:

Well, the one reaction I have about this contagion thing is that when I sit there with cancer patients and they're spitting up all these horrible things into Kleenex, I don't want to throw away their Kleenex for them. I think there are probably cells in it, and how do they get them from people to mice, and test all this stuff. It has to live somewhere, right? I don't know how crazy that is or not.

This concern may account for some of the isolation that befalls cancer patients. Most caregivers seem to be able clearly to identify thoughts they have had about their own likelihood at getting cancer. A typical reflection about this topic is:

> I sometimes think when I've got a twinge or something like that, I definitely identify first with the possibility that it could be cancer, and it definitely evokes a fear within me, and then I'll look at it and try to rationalize or rationally see what's happening.

Another provider said:

> If I thought in the back of my mind that I would catch cancer, I would be living like a banana all the time, with every little cut and bruise, and I envision myself as never dying of cancer. No one in my family ever died of cancer. They all had strokes or heart attacks or some kind of sudden death type of thing, and I always thought I would die a sudden death.

An additional comment indicates how a provider may rationalize a lack of concern about working with this patient population:

> People have asked me, "Do you think, working with cancer, that maybe you're going to get cancer? Not catch it, but just because everybody has it, think that you're going to get it, that you might program yourself for it?" I don't really think so, I think part of it is because everybody in my family died with heart problems, so I think that when I die I'll probably die of a heart attack. I don't know. I don't really worry about it. I've always been healthy, and no one in my family has had cancer, so that's part of it. I really believe there are definite familial tendencies. I guess in a way I feel a little protected.

Working with Cancer Patients and Families

Once oncology caregivers go beyond instrumental interventions and became involved with the patient's psychological responses, emotional response becomes an important issue to examine. Adequate empirical studies of the impact of working with cancer patients on caretakers do not yet exist (Shady 1976), though professionals who care for patients with life-threatening illness certainly experience strong affective reactions as a result of their work. A number of studies have indicated that physicians and nurses perceive terminal illness as extremely threatening and typically prefer to avoid death-related thoughts and feelings (Pearlman et al. 1969). Yet such avoidance, if excessive, can lead to problems in relating and responding in inappropriate ways, or can lead to a sense of professional inadequacy, helplessness, and depression (Bugen 1979; Maslach 1979; Weisman 1970). Professional and cultural guidelines that dictate suppression of emotions and idealize objectivity can create conflict for the provider who must confront his/her own humanity in the course of daily work. For example, should the provider cry with patients? Different providers express different attitudes toward this. Some providers can be closely and warmly involved with patients but feel it is not appropriate to cry with them:

> Sometimes I cry when I feel real heavy-duty stress, like with one particular family. When I got home the night after seeing them and knowing I was going to have to go back, I cried for a while because it's draining, but when I'm with people who are in an acute crisis, I think they can sense my empathy without my having to cry with them, and I don't want them to feel like I'm falling apart or that they need to take care of me, so I try to contain myself. If I experience a lot of distress about it, I take it elsewhere. I made phone calls to people that night to talk about it.

Others find it works for them sometimes to express such feelings:

> I remember the first time that I allowed myself to cry in front of parents when a child died, and that worked at that point. I felt it. I couldn't keep from crying, but I wasn't ashamed and I wasn't embarrassed, and I didn't think I was unprofessional, but I wouldn't cry with everybody. I wouldn't want to. So I'm not sure . . . you can still cry, and you can still laugh, and still be professional.

Like so many questions in this area, there is no answer about what is right or wrong. It is generally felt, however, that the meaningfulness and impact of staff interventions with patients and their families are dependent on genuine professional involvement. The therapeutic boundaries designed for traditional psychotherapy are constantly questioned by staff working in oncology settings. As stated earlier in this book, cancer patients are not psychiatric patients, thus there is the potential for newly defined staff–patient relationships. With each intervention or behavior, the caregiver opens up certain possibilities with the patient and closes off others. There is always a balance and tradeoff in saying or doing anything with patients.

Talking to patients about death can also be a stressful issue and verbal avoidance of this area in one way caregivers have of protecting themselves (Schultz and Aderman 1976). Kastenbaum (1967) found that over 80% of nurses he studied avoided responses to patients' statements regarding death. Similar findings about difficulties in working with patients with life-threatening illness have been published regarding doctors' responses (Oken 1961; Scurry et al. 1979). Unfortunately, such behavior can lead to feelings by the patients of being isolated. One of the most challenging moments for the provider is described by one clinician as follows:

> I guess realistically the most challenging moment is when someone asks, "Am I going to die?" I guess that's the hardest. I feel this tremendous sense of responsibility for having been the one they asked. I'd really rather push it off on somebody else. A typical nursing response would probably be, "Ask your doctor," or something like that. I also know that it took them a long time to work up to asking me that. I usually say, "What have they told you about that?" or "What do you think about that." And usually they'll say that they already know the answer. Sometimes I'll just come out directly and say, "Yes, everybody's going to die sometime," something to the effect that we don't know when your time will be, but we know that the cancer will probably cause your death, where somebody else will have a stroke or something like that.

In addition to verbal avoidance, caretakers physically avoid dying patients as their condition worsens (Kastenbaum and Aisenberg 1972; Livingston and Zimet 1965). The issue of distance versus closeness is one that each clinician must face. It seems that (as described in other sections) the personal involvement with patients is one of the aspects of this work that providers cite as making it all worthwhile. Again, psychodynamically trained clinicians are usually warned in their training against personal involvement and revelations. At times, however, crossing such boundaries may be the key to a patient who is feeling isolated:

> I remember the first time that I got "personal" and it was with a very belligerent, hostile, big hunk of a man, who stormed

into my office and said, "Can you make sure that my kid's going to live?" And I said, "I can't, but maybe the doctors can talk to you about that." And I asked him where he came from, and he said, "It doesn't matter." And I said, "Well, you have an Italian name, and you have an accent, so I wonder if you recently came to this country." And he said, "Yes, and I come from a town you never heard of." And I said, "Oh." And he said, "Where do you come from?" And I said, "Well, my family comes from Provincia DeLuca." And he just sort of sparked. That's an area near Florence, and he came from the town just down the mountain from that my mother's family came from. From that point on, we were able to work with him. Now I don't say this should be done all the time, but there is a time and a place for breaking down the professional barriers.

At times, when first contacting a patient, the patient may say in a somewhat angry tone, "How can you help me or understand me; you have never had cancer and don't know what it's like?" When a clinician hears such a remark from a patient, it is important to determine the underlying issue. In this case, the inexperienced clinician may respond, "Well, as a matter of fact, you're right that I don't have cancer, but a close relative of mine had it and I know what it's about." Or, "You're right about that, but I've been working in the field a long time and have a lot of experience working with cancer patients so I feel I do understand something about it." Such responses are merely superficial and miss the point that the patient feels cut off and unreachable. A more appropriate response would be, "I guess you're feeling that no one can understand what you're going through." Such a response usually does not produce a rejoinder of anger, but rather the empathic confirmation of the patient's situation usually switches the context into more productive dialogue.

There is a certain amount of unpredictability in how the caregiver's task is viewed. What some people find impossible, others find the most satisfying. For example, one clinician reports being unable to work with children:

> I never worked with children that well. I think part of it is that I like to be able to relate to somebody who understands what I'm saying, and I don't have any children of my own, so maybe I'm not really aware of just how much they know or don't know. I feel kind of lost with them. I just don't know at what age they should be understanding what things. So that's probably why. And I guess I can't handle it, if I have to give

them an injection; to adults you can explain why. To a child
you can, but for some reason, I have this thing in my mind that
it doesn't matter, they're going to cry anyway, and that bothers
me.

When asked about working with children, another clinician responded:

> I've always liked them. They're honest; they tell it like it is,
> they're direct, they're more apt to hear what is being told.
> They're not sophisticated. Oh, they do their blocking too, but
> in a blunter way. You can ask a question and know you're go-
> ing to get an answer. I remember one youngster from the ward
> on rounds, and I said, "Hi, Diane, how are you?" She replied
> directly, "Well, I'm sick or I wouldn't be here." I learned a lot
> from that answer, and I never ask how a patient in the hospital
> is anymore. . . . I think some of the youngsters have gotten
> more out of life and given more to life in five or six years than
> many of us in a lifetime, a normal lifetime.

Many individuals who work with adult cancer patients say that
they would never be emotionally capable of working with a sick
child. On the other hand, many staff involved in pediatric oncology feel they would have great difficulty working with adults. It is
apparent that individual staff, based on experience and professional training, will select the population that best suits their personal and professional needs. One cannot say that any population
of cancer patients is "easier" or "more difficult" to work with
than the other. Each can provide the highs and lows and challenges that can make staff feel positive about the roles they can
play in good patient care.

Job Meaning

Despite the stresses and apparently unsolvable problems that can
face the caregiver, many people find working in this field quite
gratifying. Some perceive the greater opportunity than in many
settings to become involved with patients in a meaningful way:

> I like working with one person at a time. I really hate being
> a charge nurse and having 40 patients, and you don't really get

to know anyone of them. I really like that one-on-one type of relationship.

When asked whether such one-to-one working relationships
could create undue strain, one nurse said:

> No, because to me it really makes my job, it makes my work
> more meaningful. I mean, not to sound corny about it, that it
> really gives it some meaning.

For many clinicians, confirmation of meaningful links with patients and their families frequently involves some follow-up contact:

> I think we do make impact on peoples' lives because a lot of
> times the family, a daughter or a husband, will actually call us
> and tell us the day that the relative died. I mean that takes a lot,
> I think. I don't know whether, if I had a relative who died, I
> would call some hospital personnel unless I felt they really cared
> about that person. It doesn't just happen to me, it happens to
> the nurses in our clinic. It just kind of reinforces our job. It
> makes up feel satisfied with it. It's not just a bunch of paper-
> work.

Social System Variables

It has generally been assumed that the major determinant of stress
for the oncology clinician is the primary task of working with life-
threatening illness in dying patients. However, an alternative
view, born out of discussions with caregivers and research, is that
social system variables have a significant influence on stress, attitudes, morale, and patient care behavior (Mohl 1981). One experienced provider in looking at those who do not last in the field observed:

> People who have left this work have left stressed, but it was
> outside stress, not the stress of the work they were doing
> but of pressures from administration, directors, physicians, co-
> workers.

The kinds of social system variables that influence the experience and coping of the cancer caregiver include relationships with
authority, covert group values and norms, peer relationships, and
division of labor. The unique blend of responsibility and emo-

tional closeness to patients in the context of professional isolation can be especially toxic. One nurse reflected:

> The doctor comes and the doctor leaves, but the nurse is there with the patient and the family all the time. Patients confide, oftentime, things that they won't confide to the physician, and it becomes very frustrating for a nurse, because the nurse has no place to go in that period. A nurse cannot dictate authority as a way of coping and removing herself from the stress, and the nurse is kind of stuck in the middle of everything. She has no place to go.

Such a situation is especially likely to occur in this field since the psychosocial dimensions of oncology programs are thinly staffed and there is a high probability that a nurse or social worker will be functioning in isolation. Furthermore, home care providers and visiting nurses are often isolated from peer groups by the decentralized nature of their work. In addition, such home care agencies are not usually budgeted to provide time for staff meetings that could furnish a setting for sharing of cases and peer support.

Physicians have their own risk of isolation as many practice alone or do not have the opportunity to ventilate feelings associated with their work. A significant contribution to the high incidence of suicide and substance abuse among physicians comes from participation in a system in which there is little opportunity simply to be a person who hurts, as opposed to the God-like professional who has to have all the answers. One physician reflected on the opportunity to relate to other providers that he found as a member of a hospice program, but which had been lacking before:

> By and large, in a professional sense, I am blessed by being a part of a hospice. It has expanded what I am and has leavened out potentially a lot of stresses that I think I do face and would otherwise face. It really has enabled me to sort of hear myself, as if on a tape recorder, by hearing feedback to me by people I know care about me, and are sharing the same kinds of stresses, those comments that I have offered. It gives me a very appropriate and I think realistic sense of what is truly real and what is not. I think that physicians lack that. I think it's easy to believe that we are very good, that we are really right most of the time. I think many physicians know that they are not right, and I think how they handle those stresses, contributes in a large part

to how successful they are in warding off their own impending crisis.

What, from a social system perspective, helps clinicians in some settings function more effectively and under less distress than clinicians in other settings, even when the task is the same? This is an important question to consider as clinicians who are having problems may blame themselves, and feel inadequate and frustrated, as if they were bad or incompetent professionals, when, in fact, the problem may lie outside themselves. All clinicians should develop a systems perspective as a part of a repertoire of assessing their own clinical problems. One study (Mohl et al. 1982) has assessed the assumptions that social system variables determine nurses' stress and attitudes by comparing the work attitudes and clinical distress of nurses on two general medical units and two medical intensive care units. It turned out that one intensive care unit had much lower levels of clinical stress in the staff than any of the other units. This unit was characterized by having significantly better staff (defined as the degree to which supervisors supported workers and encouraged mutual support). The nursing care coordinator on that unit treated her staff as responsible, competent professionals who were to be listened to with respect. It was open acknowledgment of the stressful nature of the work with much encouragement from mutual support. Such support by supervising staff, rather than peer cohesion, work pressure, or unit type, emerged as the variable that distinguished the low-distress unit. Support groups to accomplish this end have been described (Mohl 1980; Weiner and Caldwell, 1981).

In many settings, a less formal supportive process occurs as a result of the program structure. One provider commented on what she felt supportive about her work setting:

> I think there are protections within how this department works from having it be too overwhelming, and I think those have to do with a lot of other things to do besides 100% direct patient care. I think that would be way too much. I think the meetings are helpful, and I think that, with the patient with whom I spent the last two days helping her through her husband's death, the fact that so many people were aware that that was going on was supportive to me, even if I didn't have a lot of direct contact, I felt kind of supported by the whole system, and the staff was really good.

It has been suggested that group support would be useful for cancer center personnel to lessen their sense of failure and discouragement in the face of the unrelenting stress of caring for cancer patients. This recommendation has been made even though little objective evidence exists that documents the effectiveness of group therapy for this population.

Group process has been used for training oncology fellows (Artiss and Levine 1973; Wise 1977). Both these groups were basically educative in nature and dealt neither with group process nor psychotherapy issues. Other articles on insight-promoting groups have been methodologically inadequate to confirm results (Yano 1977; Van Ostenberg 1973; Sainsbury and Milton, 1975; Wodinsky 1974; Janes and Weise, 1970).

It is increasingly recognized that there are risks involved in participating in groups in that the experience may be as damaging for some as it is beneficial for others (Galinsky and Schopler 1977). To investigate part of this question, Silberfarb and Levine (1980) assessed the attitudes of oncology nurses to job-related concepts prior to and following six months of weekly 1½-hour psychodynamically oriented support group sessions. These attitudes were compared with those of oncology nurses not in the group experience during the same time span. It turned out that the nurses who had completed the group experience showed more negative attitude shifts to work and a greater attitude change in the negative direction than those not in the group. These findings suggest that a group situation in which individuals are encouraged to bring up and discuss personal work-related problems in an open-ended way may not be an effective means for assisting individuals coping with the stresses of being a provider or in improving patient care. The importance of maintaining denial on the part of caregivers must always be respected, as it is with patients. Over all, the author of that study suggests that an educational model may be more appropriate for oncology providers. This educational model is presently used in many centers with encouraging results.

Conclusions

Caregivers working in an oncology setting face many interesting, challenging, and difficult professional and personal dilemmas. Although "outsiders" will often respond by asking "How do you do it?" many oncology staff remain in the field for relatively long periods of their careers. Like many other areas, the biopsychosocial aspects of oncology have become an important subspecialty of medicine, nursing, social service, psychiatry, and psychology. As a result of major recent interest and development of progress within the last ten years, oncology is presently creating a model of care that is being implemented with other chronic and life-threatening illnesses. It is for this reason that staff development issues in oncology continue to be explored, evaluated, and documented. The oncology clinician, whether the nurse, psychologist, psychiatrist, oncologist, or social worker, is potentially an important link in developing new team approaches to the successful implementation of better comprehensive standards of care for all populations of medically ill patients (see chapter 8).

Rather than develop psychodynamically oriented groups, staff can be supported by having case presentations that are biopsychosocial in nature. For example, a series of staff group support sessions would include presentations of patient issues around physical management, psychological management, and social management, and often lend themselves to discussions about various staff members' involvement with patients and their families. This psychoeducational model provides a nonthreatening way for staff to gain a sense of mastery over the difficulties of caring for the cancer patient.

One staff member identified her key support system as follows:

> We were all of the same department, the nurses, physicians, the technicians, and it was a small group. It was based on case presentations in an informal manner. Yet we all shared the emotional traumas of working with really sick patients. It was an enormous help.

References

Artiss, K., and Levine, A. S.: Doctor–patient relationship in severe illness: A seminar for oncology fellows. *N. Engl. J. Med.* 288 (1973): 1210–1214.

Bugen, L. A.: Emotions: Their pressence and impact upon the helping role. In C. Garfield (Ed.), *Stress and survival: The emotional realities of life-threatening illness*. St. Louis: Mosby, 1979.

FREUDENBERGER, H. J.: Staff burn-out *J. Soc. Iss.* 30 (1974): 159–165.

GALINSKY, M. J., AND SCHOPLER, J. H.: Warning: Groups may be dangerous. *Soc. Work* 22 (1977): 89–94.

JANES, R. G., WEISE, A. E.: Psychiatric liaison with a cancer research center. *Comp. Psychiat.* 11 (1970): 336–345.

KASTENBAUM, R.: Multiple perspectives on a geriatric "death valley." *Commun. Ment. Health J.* 3 (1967): 21–29.

KASTENBAUM, R., AND AISENBERG, R.: *The psychology of death.* New York: Springer, 1972.

KOLOTKIN, R. A.: Preventing burn-out and reducing stress in terminal care. In Harry J. Sobel (Ed.), *Behavior therapy in terminal care.* Cambridge, Mass.: Ballinger, 1981.

LIVINGSTON, P. B., AND ZIMET, C. N.: Death anxiety, authoritarianism, and choice of specialty in medical students. *J. Nerv. Ment. Dis.* 140 (1965): 222–230.

MASLACH, C.: The burn-out syndrome and patient care. In C. Garfield (Ed.), *Stress and survival: The emotional realities of life-threatening illness.* St. Louis: Mosby, 1979.

MOHL, P. C.: Group process interpretations in liaison psychiatric nurse groups. *Gen. Hosp. Psychiat.* 2 (1980): 104–111.

————: A review of systems approaches to consultation-liaison psychiatry. *Gen. Hosp. Psychiat.* 3 (1981): 103–110.

MOHL, P. C., DENNY, N. R., MOTE, T. A., AND GOLDWATER, C.: Hospital unit stressors that affect nurses: Primary task vs social factors. *Psychosomatics* 23 (1982): 366–374.

OKEN, D.: The physician, the patient, and cancer. *Ill. Med. J.* 120 (1961): 333–334.

PARSONS, T.: Social structure and dynamic process: the case of modern medical practice. In *The social system.* New York: Free Press, 1951, chapter 10.

PEARLMAN, J., STOTSKY, B., AND DOMINICK, J.: Attitudes toward death among nursing home personnel. *J. Genet. Psychol.* 114: 63–75, 1969.

SAINSBURY, M. J., AND MILTON, G. W.: The nurse in a cancer ward. *Med. J. Austr.* 2 (1975): 911–913.

SCHULTZ, R., AND ADERMAN, D.: How the medical staff copes with dying patients: A critical review. *Omega* 7 (1976): 11–21.

SCURRY, M. I., BRUHN, J. G., AND BUNCE, H.: The house officer and the dying patient: Attitudes, experiences and needs. *Gen. Hosp. Psychiat.* 1 (1979): 301–305.

SHADY, G.: Death anxiety and care of the terminally-ill: A review of the clinical literature. *Can. Psychol. Rev.* 17 (1976): 137–142.

SILBERFARB, P., AND LEVINE, P.: Psychosocial aspects of neoplastic disease. *Gen. Hosp. Psychiat.* 3 (1980): 192–197.

VACHON, M. L.: Staff stress in care of the terminally ill. Qual. Rev. Bull. (1979) 13–17.

VAN OSTENBERG, D. L.: Therapy groups for staff and interns. *Hosp. Commun. Psychiat.* 24 (1973): 474–475.

WEINER, M. F., AND CALDWELL, T.: Stresses and coping in ICU nursing: II. The nurse group. *Gen. Hosp. Psychiat.* 3 (1981): 129–134.

WEISMAN, A.: Misgivings and misconceptions in the psychiatric care of terminal patients. *Psychiatry* 33 (1970): 67–81.

WISE, T. N.: Utilization of group process in training oncology fellows. *Int. J. Group Psychother.* 27 (1977): 105–111.

WODINSKY, A.: Psychiatric consultation with nurses on a leukemia service. *Ment. Hyg.* 48 (1974): 282–287.

YANO, B. S.: What about us? *J. Pract. Nurs.* 27 (1977): 28–38.

CHAPTER 8

Psychosocial Oncology: The Multidisciplinary Team Approach

IN RECENT YEARS , increasing attention to the psychiatric and psychosocial needs of cancer patients has led to the collaborative involvement of psychiatrists and other mental health professionals in many oncology treatment programs. Because such collaboration is relatively new, there remains much confusion as to exactly what work needs to be done and by whom. Among the most commonly heard questions and concerns that need to be addressed are:

1. How should patients who need to see a mental health professional be identified?
2. What problems are commonly encountered in arranging for such consultation?
3. What are the unique contributions of the psychiatrist, social worker, nurse, and psychologist, and what clinical areas do they share?

Problems in Identification and Referral of Patients to Mental Health Team Members

Many oncology programs without a formal psychiatric consultation-liaison component have a variety of support services and re-

194

habilitative programs already in place (Blumberg and Flaherty 1980; Harvey 1982). At a minimum, patients and their families are being informed about what resources are available, what they offer, and how to become involved with them should they wish to do so (NIH Publication no. 80–2080, 1980). However, when mental health professionals are specifically associated with an oncology program, it may not be clear to the oncology staff, or to the mental health professionals themselves, as to how, when, and to whom referrals should be made.

It is well known that there is a significant incidence of misdiagnosis of psychiatric disorders in oncology patients (Levine et al. 1978). As detailed in chapter 4, a plethora of medical disorders masquerade as psychological or behavioral problems. There seems to be a significant underrecognition of both psychiatric and psychosocial problems by physicians (Steinberg et al. 1980). The incidence of depression, especially, appears to be generally underestimated by oncologists, and when it is suspected, its differential diagnosis is usually overlooked (Goldberg 1981). When depression is identified, it is often inadequately treated (Derogatis et al. 1979). Insufficient treatment of pain presents another challenge for many patients (Angell 1982). A high proportion of medical and surgical inpatients experience emotional difficulties related to their illnesses or medical care. Yet, while psychiatric morbidity has been found in 30 to 60% of general hospital inpatients, and the prevalence of psychiatric disorders among cancer patients has been put at 47%, only 1 to 13% are referred for psychiatric evaluation (Lipowski 1967; Kligerman and McKegney 1971; Derogatis et al. 1983).

Physicians' tolerance of distress in patients can be quite high, and a psychiatric consultation may be avoided unless the patient's behavior grossly disrupts medical care or creates excessive uncertainty (Meyer and Mendelson 1961). A number of factors are probably responsible for physician resistance to recognizing emotional factors in patients.

It may be difficult for many physicians to relinquish their sense of control and autonomy over patient care. The special relationship developed with patients with life-threatening disorders is intense and can tend to become exclusive. Other consultants can be seen as intruders. To some physicians, the need for a mental health consultant implies that they are not the "complete" physician. Resentment over intrusion into the doctor–patient relationship is especially likely if a referral is made by a nurse, technician, or social worker who bypasses the physician. Anyone in contact with the patient who feels that a psychiatric consultation is indicated should raise the issue, and the data to support it, to the primary physician.

In other instances, the need to maintain emotional equilbrium may require emotional distancing from the patient and, therefore, lead to denial of the patient's profound emotional reaction to life-threatening illness. This denial can be bolstered by the unsupported belief that the psychiatrist could not be of help to a patient with life-threatening illness since many of these problems are an unavoidable and expectable part of the illness. Many oncologists have stereotypic ideas about what psychiatrists and other mental health professionals do. "They just talk . . . they upset people more . . . they don't understand anything about cancer patients." Such concerns often seem to be confirmed by poor experiences with psychiatrists who were not specialists in working at the medical interface with this population. However, in the review by Steinberg et al. (1980) of 50 cases of patients for whom the physician had resisted psychiatric consultation, the physicians' reasons for not obtaining a consultation were not accurate in virtually every one of the patients seen and almost every patient was helped by the consultation.

Some of the discomfort with suggesting mental health referral arises because of the concern that the idea might offend, anger, or stigmatize the patient. Such fears have, in fact, been shown to be unrealistic in the great majority of patients who were interviewed following the suggestion that they have a psychiatric consultation, but before the actual referral (Schwab 1971). In fact, more than 80% of the patients interviewed by Schwab responded favorably to the suggestion of consultation, whether or not they were actually referred. There obviously needs to be more discussion between psychiatrists and oncologists as to what to say when making a referral. There is concern that the patient will react negatively: "Are you saying that I'm mentally disturbed?" or "I think you're the one with poor judgment, not me." It is important for the referring professional to discuss the reasons for and purpose of the referral to validate its significance in the patient's overall care as well as to provide some perspective for the patient. The oncologist should be encouraged to cultivate a straightforward style of communicating the need for referral. In cases where there seems to be a special patient sensitivity to this area, referrals to a nonpsychiatric member of the mental health team (for example, a social worker or nurse clinician) may be a more productive road to take. However, this arrangement can place social workers or nurses in a somewhat awkward situation if there is a feeling of having to disguise the purpose of the evaluation or their own identity. Generally, a patient can be engaged most easily by creating a focus on some specific jointly acknowledged problem such as pain, financial concerns, or difficulty in managing some complexities of the treatment system.

The lack of role definition of members of the psychiatric team adds to referral problems. Even after a need to make a referral is perceived, lack of clarity about what to expect only adds to the ambiguity and to the anxiety of patient and provider.

It is clear that the oncology staff cannot always be expected to recognize or make appropriate psychiatric referrals. Therefore, there is a need for a psychiatric liaison team member to participate in the oncology program. Integration of mental health consultation cannot be accomplished by writing a memo stating its availability, setting a policy, or providing occasional consultation. Such consultation can raise basic issues of what is involved in patient care and, therefore, requires a gradual and ongoing process of interaction among the professional participants (Brodsky 1970). Obviously, it may not be warranted, cost effective, or even possible to have all distressed cancer patients seen by a mental health professional. A concerned physician, sensitive medical technician, oncology nurse, or clinical social worker can provide support sufficient to the needs of many patients. This implies the necessity for the mental health team to furnish ongoing liaison with these groups to help them develop skills in this area and to learn when and to whom to refer. At times, when the medical treatment staff is not aware of the need for mental health referral, the patient or family may be.

While any of the professionals could provide this liaison function, we believe there is some advantage in having a psychiatric social worker in this position. Underlying psychosocial problems often present as medical issues and somatic preoccupations (Barsky 1979; Rosen et al. 1972). When the symptoms of patients are thought not to be medically warranted, a referral is often made to the social worker, though sometimes not before excessive and unnecessary medical testing. Furthermore, medical staff often perceives concrete needs as being the main issue involved in distressed patients. Although concrete services are the most frequent kind of referral to a social worker, it is clear (as elaborated in the following sections) that many of these cases have underlying psychiatric or psychosocial problems. The disadvantage of having a psychiatrist as liaison is that some professionals and patients feel less comfortable with a ''shrink'' than with a less stigmatized social worker. Further, the concrete service referrals would probably not be made to the psychiatrist, but would be shuttled off to be processed by a nonpsychiatric social worker who would be more likely to miss the clinical issue involved.

The psychiatric liaison person must attend, on a regular basis, the clinical staff meetings of the oncology program. Such ongoing contact is basic to successful liaison as it prevents misunderstandings of roles and legitimizes the inclusion of the liaison person as a core member of the team. Further, when the liaison person functions in isolation rather than through frequent face-to-face contacts with the medical clinicians, it often turns out that the written reasons for referral do not represent the actual underlying concerns that the medical clinicians have for making the referral. Seeing patients on the basis of information from referral forms alone can be a dangerous business, unless one believes that ''real'' reasons will be given in medical referrals, an expectation that is unrealistic. Further, one cannot always rely on the patient to provide the reason for referral. Providing accurate written referral requests seems unfeasible as it would require more writing. Also, it often involves feelings of conflict on the part of the medical referrer, who may be uncomfortable or unwilling to put information viewed as personal or potentially damaging on a public piece of paper. At other times, the clinician may hesitate to put in writing information that reflects the feelings of the provider him/herself (e.g., ''I don't like this patient''). Having the liaison person talk to the referrer is important not only for finding out what actually is taking place, but also as a means of becoming integrated with the clinic team.

The Multidisciplinary Team

Multidisciplinary has been defined as members of diverse disciplines in the same setting interacting informally. The concept of the team, however, implies a more coordinated arrangement that some people have called interdisciplinary (Bloom and Parad 1976). Coordination of mental health professionals in an interdisciplinary team has been endorsed by psychiatrists (Kaltreider et al. 1974; Lipowski 1979), social workers (Bergman and Fritz 1982; Ell and Morrison 1981; Lee 1980; Lewis et al. 1976) and nurses (Barton and Kelso 1971; Burch and Meredith 1974; Holstein and Schwab 1965).

The concept of the multidisciplinary team does not exist simply because there are four professions (psychiatry, psychology, nursing, and social work) all competing for overlapping territory and role functions. When the unique contributions of team members have not been thought through, it is often the case that there is an excess of competitiveness, strained feelings, political hostility, and confusion that finally impacts negatively on patient care. While it is true that a number of clinical functions overlap disciplines, it is by understanding the unique contribution of each team member that an effective and logical clinical force becomes created.

By way of an introductory overview, the Psychiatric-Oncology Consultation Team at Rhode Island Hospital is a subdivision of the Division of Consultation-Liaison of the Department of Psychiatry. This division was formed to consolidate knowledge, skills, and attitudes needed by a variety of professionals to deal with oncology consultations requested of our program. Its organization also implies that the Department of Psychiatry takes overall responsibility for the standards for clinical practice, though representatives of each profession participating are expected to function as autonomous clinical professionals. Members of the team include two psychiatrists, two doctoral-level psychologists, two master's-level social workers, and a nurse-clinical specialist. Patients are referred by radiation, medical, orthopedic, and pediatric oncology services. Members of our team, in addition to performing oncology consultations, participate in psychosocial oncology research and also provide some consultation to nononcology services. The team forms the core of psychiatric-oncology rounds, which are held weekly and are attended by oncologists, visiting and home care nurses, hospice workers, and other mental health professionals who deal with cancer patients. This meeting provides a crucial link for diverse professions that are otherwise administratively unrelated and an opportunity to help individuals get to know each other and thus break down barriers that can interfere with coordinating patient care. General consultation case review rounds take place twice each week and are available for review of individual case problems. These meetings are independent of an in addition to attendance by members of this team at the clinical rounds held by oncology services themselves. The team members have done approximately 481 evaluations and 1600 follow-up visits over the past year. In their liaison capacities, team members interact with the medical staff both in multidisciplinary conferences on topics such as pain control or depression and in meetings with oncologists and staff to deal with the stresses of providing care to cancer patients.

The Biopsychosocial Data Base

For the multidisciplinary team to work, some sort of data base format must be developed so that the nonmedical mental health clinician can gather information appropriate to a biopsychosocial evaluation and begin to identify, in a systematic way, patients who require services from other team members. To make this possible, the clinician must be integrated into a psychiatric team that has adequate representation by a biomedically oriented psychiatrist who is in a position to make diagnostic assessments of cases seen by other team members. This input is especially critical given the high incidence of medical disorders that masquerade as psychosocial problems (see chapter 4). Some program descriptions of liaison with oncology programs do not adequately emphasize the medical component of the psychiatric liaison person (Capone et al. 1979; Small and Mitchell 1979).

The process of adaptation to cancer takes place at the confluence of biologic, psychological, and social systems. Physical symptoms alone do not account for the distress of the cancer patient, nor does the presentation of seemingly psychological or social complaint assure that an underlying medical disorder is not a direct or aggravating cause. Patients with unrecognized psychiatric disorders are often referred to nonpsychiatric clinicians and the role of medical factors in psychosocial distress is often not adequately appreciated by the physician. Koranyi (1979) has documented that social workers are almost universally unaware of underlying medical disorders relevant to the psychological or social symptoms being evaluated. This implies that the oncology social worker, nurse, or psychologist should be trained to recognize such problems. To become a colleague on a team of professionals involved in psychosocial oncology, the nonpsychiatrist must be prepared to speak the language of the biomedical as well as the psychosocial disciplines, must be aware of those medical disorders that present as psychological symptoms, and must learn to conceptualize patient problems in a biopsychosocial model. The biopsychosocial data base is the fundamental clinical tool needed to assure a systematic approach to such patient care. Without such a data base, it is too easy for the clinician to make assumptions about the etiology of a patient's problems according to his/her particular bias or predisposition.

The biomedical knowledge necessary to use this data base does not require that the social worker or nurse become a "minipsychiatrist." Instead, the intent is to augment the traditional knowledge base of the nonpsychiatrist with information necessary for him/her to become significant contributor to the multidisciplinary oncology team.

The data base is not an end in itself, but a means to an end. It is not meant to be used as rigid outline which that be filled out sequentially at the risk of alienating the patient and destroying the therapeutic relationship. As one becomes familiar with its contents, it is not difficult to gather all the appropriate information in the course of a clinical interview that remains sensitive to interpersonal nuances. The contents of this data base represent information that a majority of the competent clinicians routinely gather in some fashion during every evaluation. The particular order of the questions and the format are somewhat arbitrary, and the inclusion or omission of some items can serve as the basis for constructive revision. However, when one takes up the task of organizing and writing a data base within certain time and space limitations, decisions about what to include or exclude have to be made. This particular data base (see the appendix B) remains a living document that is altered as warranted by growing clinical experience of its usefulness in a particular setting. Since a clinician's time is so limited, he/she should understand the purpose of every question asked and should feel that each question has a potential to alter further clinical decisions about the patient. A more complete exposition of the data base has been written for the nonpsychiatrist by Wallace and associates (in press).

A systematized data base simultaneously serves a number of needs in the oncology setting. It facilitates communication among a variety of disciplines by organizing information into an identifiable format that becomes familiar to the staff. Too often, information obtained in a psychosocial interview is organized in idiosyncratic ways, is illegible, or has significant errors of omission or commission that make the clinical effort much less useful to the rest of the treatment team. Further, since patients in oncology settings may be seen longitudinally by different providers, this format establishes a true data base that lends itself to the problem-oriented record keeping that is increasingly a part of health care. Naturally, patients do not need a new data base for each visit. Once a good data base has been established, the need for only minor revisions rather than complete review actually saves clinician time in the long run. Finally, the data base serves not only as a uniform approach to patient evaluation, but also becomes an important teaching tool that can be used interchangeably by a variety of disciplines.

Some clinicians may feel that asking questions that review medical and psychiatric history may be intrusive, may impair the therapeutic relationship with the patient, or may be irrelevant to the concern of helping cancer patients who are distressed. The time and place for such a data base are not always agreed upon, and there are times when sections of it may be inappropriate. However, we feel that no patient can be understood apart from a context that includes significant medical, psychological, and social events. Patients in distress are looking, above all, for a competent and caring clinician. Caring itself is important, but the professional adds another dimension by conveying that the apparently chaotic and overwhelming distress of the patient can be organized, understood, and managed. While clinicians must develop their own style to obtain a data base, there are basic elements that most good clinicians would include. A history of past psychiatric history should be included as such patients are probably at increased risk when distressed. There should be questions of other significant life events, since there is evidence that these are cumulative in the final coping of the patient and may be missed if there is excessive focus on the medical issue itself. The family history is important, both for its psychological and medical dimensions. People tend to feel that the experience of family members will be repeated in themselves. There should also be inclusion of the patient's medical history and habits, including alcohol and drug use, as well as current medications and drugs.

The biopsychosocial approach to patient care allows for different dimensions of problems to be present simultaneously and to interact to produce the manifest clinical picture. For example, a patient's reaction to cancer can be shaped by personality, as well as by a psychiatric diagnosis such as major depression, an organic mental disorder, a problem in the family, or some concrete social problem. The role of the mental health team member who sees such a patient should not be as an exclusionist or an isolationist, but rather as a coordinator who speaks to the interplay of the various dimensions that are woven into the patient's problem. The use of the biopsychosocial data base allows the clinician to play this critical role. It will also maximize the efficiency with which the nonpsychiatrist can interact with the psychiatric coordinator on the team. By uncovering potential problem areas through this data base, the social worker will discover areas that require further psychiatric consultation. Rather than recreating the entire data base, the psychiatric consultant can then utilize the information obtained and focus more specifically on a problem area, such as the possibility of behavioral consequences of medical drugs or the possible indication for the use of psychopharmacologic agents.

The Contributions of Different Mental Health Specialists

The Unique Contribution of the Psychiatrist

Psychiatry has experienced its own identity crisis over the past decade, passing through a broad and almost self-destructive detour consisting of an almost exclusive immersion in psychotherapy, with decreasing involvement in the world of medicine. While there has always remained a cadre of general hospital and consultation-liaison psychiatrists who maintained an interface with other medical disciplines, most of those in the field removed their white coats and withdrew from their primary identity as physicians. For a period of time in the early 1970s, psychiatry even dropped the requirement for a medical internship as part of its training and allowed medical students to enter directly into specialty training, bypassing altogether the internship experience and its associated medical identity development. Fortunately, this policy was seen as a near-tragic mistake and was reversed around 1974. Psychiatry has realized, within the past few years, that its major contribution to mental health must be drawn from its biomedical roots, with emphasis on diagnostic abilities and breadth of training that allows for a review of the interaction of both biologic and psychosocial factors in each patient.

The unique contribution of the psychiatrist is the ability to provide differential diagnosis of disorders of mood, thought, and behavior. Depression, for example, as discussed in chapter 4, cannot
be viewed as a diagnosis but rather must be considered a symptom, which, like other medical symptoms such as fever, jaundice,
or anemia, must prompt a thorough medical and psychological
evaluation. The inclination of many clinicians working with depressed cancer patients is to react with statements such as,
"Wouldn't you be depressed if you had cancer?" Such statements
too often serve as disclaimers for further careful evaluation. The
literature, however, has amply documented the high incidence of
biomedical disorders that can produce symptoms that appear as
depression. Similarly, the ability to evaluate differentially organic
mental disorders, including expertise in the behavioral awareness
of the effects of medications on the central nervous system (CNS),
is crucial to understanding many of the presumed psychological
impairments in cancer patients (see chapter 5). The knowledge of
psychopharmacology (including appropriate use of analgesics) is
also crucial to the overall management of some cancer patients
(see chapter 6). When referring a patient who has undergone
some change in personality of concern to friends or physician, the
consulting psychiatrist (who must, of course, be adequately
trained in behavioral neurology) must be able to review the medical chart, including metabolic and diagnostic tests, and understand the somatic consequences of illness and therapy. A strong
medical background is critical in the assessment and management
of pain. No other mental health profession is in a position to provide this input into the assessment of patient problems.

The medical presence of the psychiatrist as a physician on a
multidisciplinary consultation team is the cornerstone of high-
quality psychiatric consultation care to an oncology population.
The psychiatrist must be in a position to review cases interviewed
by other nonphysician members of the mental health team to assure that adequate medical input has taken place. Such case review and coordination can be facilitated by the use of a standardized psychiatric data base that allows team members of various
disciplines to gather uniformly pertinent information, which can
then be presented on a regular basis for medical review.

The data base, discussed in a previous section, makes the role
of the psychiatrist more efficient by providing input for biomedical
screening. It also implies several things that the psychiatrist is not:

The psychiatrist is not necessarily the first clinician to see the patient. The psychiatrist is not necessarily the primary therapist for the patient. The psychiatrist does not necessarily have unique expertise in the nonbiomedical dimensions of cancer patients. Actually, given the shortage of psychiatrists and the advantages that nonpsychiatric clinicians may have in certain settings, it probably would not be ideal to have psychiatry play the initial or primary role, even if funding and availability were not major issues. However, there are certain cases where the complexity of the medical disorder interacting with the psychosocial adaptation is such that the psychiatrist in fact may be the person best suited to be the primary clinician for the patient. Finally, psychiatry has some advantage in liaison with other physicians who may be more oriented to deal on a physician-to-physician level. A good liaison psychiatrist may be successful in providing an entree for other mental health services and in integrating factions that might not otherwise get together.

The Unique Contribution of the Psychologist

There has been an explosion of subspecialty areas within psychology, each developing its own training programs and requirements. Therefore, it is often not easy to evaluate the background, training experiences, or specific skills one can expect from a particular psychologist. Among the various "subspecialties" are counseling, educational, rehabilitation, industrial, experimental, social, and child developmental psychologies. Furthermore, there has been the development of more clinically oriented psychotherapy training programs that have dropped the requirement for a research dissertation and grant a psychology doctorate (Psy.D.) degree, but not a doctor of philosophy (Ph.D.) degree in psychology. Some psychologists are heavily steeped in research methodology, including such areas as statistical analysis of social science research; others are more clinically oriented, though within clinical work there are a variety of approaches. These include behavioral, psychodynamic, rehabilitative, and counseling. In addition, there are psychologists whose work heavily immerses them in the area of psychophysiology. Recently there has been a mushrooming development of a field known as "behavioral medicine," and an appli-

cation of its principles to populations including terminal patients
(H. Sobel 1981). While a definition of this term has not been uniformly accepted, the field concerns itself with the application of
behavioral science knowledge to the field of medicine; it includes,
but is not limited to, applying behavior therapy to medical patients. The growing popularity of this area has led to increasing involvement of psychologists in the medical care system. Psychologists with a behavioral medicine background and orientation have
brought with them unique skills of significant benefit to patients.

Such psychologists are specifically trained to provide behavioral interventions, including self-regulatory therapies (relaxation
and biofeedback) and behavior modification. Such skills are pertinent to a large number of specific situations with cancer patients,
including the reduction of pain associated with complications of
the disease or with repetitive adverse procedures, such as chemotherapy and bone marrow biopsies (Burish and Lyles 1980; Turk
and Rennert 1981). It is now clear that certain responses, such as
nausea and vomiting or extreme anxiety, in some cases can be
classically conditioned and therefore are amenable to behavioral
intervention (Nesse et al. 1980) (see chapter 5). In addition, the
anorexia that often accompanies chemotherapy, and which can
lead to profound nutritional impairment and debilitation, sometimes can be corrected by a behavioral approach as it has become
established as a conditioned response to treatment (Bernstein
1978). As such interventions can make a significant difference in
the medical status of the patient, it is crucial that one member of
the team have these skills. Generally, but not necessarily, that
member will be the team psychologist who is trained in a behavioral medicine model.

One of the major issues facing the cancer patient is loss of control. In a sense, the patient realizes that his/her very cells are out
of control. Further, the patient is regularly exposed to high-tech-
nology interventions that contribute to a sense of helplessness.
The depression that accompanies cancer sometimes can be con-
ceptualized in terms of a learned helplessness model in which the
patient thinks, "Nothing I do matters anyway, so why try?"
Therefore, when introduced as an adjunct in pain control or in the
management of excessive anxiety, self-regulatory techniques (such
as muscle relaxation, meditation, or biofeedback) can be an important means of giving the patient a sense of mastery over his/her
own body (W. K. Sobel 1981).

The direct and indirect effects of cancer on the CNS can be profound (see chapter 4). Direct invasion of the brain by tumor or metastasis can often present as a psychological disorder. The effect of chemotherapy and radiation on brain function is an area currently under investigation (see chapter 5). As a result of an increasing awareness of the CNS effects of cancer and its treatments, it may be important to delineate the neuropsychiatric impairments as part of a comprehensive patient evaluation. Neuropsychiatric testing is a specialized form of psychological testing designed to assess the functional integrity of the brain. It differs from what many people think of as classical psychological testing, which often includes projective procedures such as the Rorschach (inkblot) test. Neuropsychological testing often includes procedures such as fine motor coordination, visual–spatial integration, perceptual function, abstract reasoning, attention, and concentration. Skilled neuropsychological testers can tell, with a high degree of certainty, whether some apparent psychological difficulty is actually caused by impairment of the brain as a result of some medical disorder. In many cases, this testing can localize the region of the brain involved. Such testing procedures are often administered by first using a screening battery, which may take about 90 minutes, to determine whether more extensive testing procedures, which can take about four hours, are actually necessary. The following case illustrates the significant contribution that a neuropsychologist can make in clinical care:

> A 40-year-old white male presented at the emergency room following a generalized seizure. A computerized axial tomography (CAT) scan showed a large tumor located deep in the left side of his brain, which was further defined with an arteriogram. He was placed on anticonvulsants and a steroid to reduce inflammation and was released from the hospital for further outpatient evaluation. Because of the deep location of the tumor, the patient was treated primarily with radiation, since an attempt to biopsy the tumor could have led to some permanent loss of speech and other motor abilities. Following completion of radiation therapy, he continued to have intermittent focal seizures. Two months later, a repeat CAT scan showed no evidence of the previously noted tumor mass. Repeated physical examination and laboratory studies, including endocrine evaluation, were normal. Everyone involved was highly gratified at the treatment response and assumed that the pa-

tient had some form of highly radiosensitive tumor. The patient and family returned home filled with hopeful expectations about recovering their normal way of life. However, the patient was never the same—he tried to go back to work (as an electrical engineer) but would come home early, and after several weeks refused to continue despite the initial encouragement and eventual insistence by the family. Because of his lack of motivation and irritability at home, despite little objective neurological deficit, he was referred for psychiatric evaluation with a presumed depression.

On initial evaluation, the patient acknowledged decreased interest in his usual activities, concentration and memory difficulties, decreased libido, and fatigue. When asked why he could not seem to get back to work, he said that the circuit boards he worked on no longer seemed to make sense. He tried for a while, but began to feel so frustrated that he wanted to avoid work. During the interview, it was somewhat difficult to get the patient to elaborate on what he said, and his wife began to take a more active role. She began to express her frustration with his "bad attitude" about things. She began to describe her difficulty in sitting by while her husband just "let himself go." When the patient began to stare out of the window, his wife quickly pointed out such behavior as a perfect example of how he was not facing up to his problem, and how every time she tried to talk seriously about these things he would withdraw and apparently refuse to face the issues before them. When asked about this, the patient said he was not sure what they had just been talking about; he went on to say that he was intermittently discouraged but not hopeless, and had no suicidal ideation. He reported no problems with sleeping or appetite. He had no previous personal or family psychiatric history. He did not use alcohol or other drugs. Because of the psychiatric concern about his impaired cognitive function, neuropsychological evaluation was performed.

Results of neuropsychiatric testing (Halstead–Reitan battery) indicated that a dramatic decrease in his intellectual ability had taken place. He was having considerable difficulty with his immediate memory, concentration, attention span, information recall, and visual–spatial organization. Results of testing suggested definite bilateral organic involvement, possibly due to the initial tumor, the radiation, or both.

Uncovering this patient's neuropsychiatric deficits had important implications for understanding and managing his symptoms. It was explained to his wife that exhorting the patient to "snap out of it" served only to frustrate him further.

His reluctance to adapt to his new situation was not psychological "resistance," but the result of an impairment involving information integration and planning. His lack of motivation to return to work was an outcome of frustration with his inability to perform specialized tasks such as "troubleshooting" electrical circuits. The testing allowed the clinician to help the patient stop seeing himself as a weak, "bad" person who was somehow failing to live up to what was expected of him as a good patient. It allowed his wife to stop pushing him because of her own somewhat misdirected, though well-intentioned, concern that he work toward recovery. It allowed the clinician to limit the time of the sessions to a period more appropriate to the patient's attention span and to shift from an abstract psychodynamic model (with an emphasis on the psychological meaning of events) to a rehabilitative model (with an emphasis on making the most of the patient's intact skills and avoiding the frustration and secondary despair that emerge from unrealistic therapeutic expectations). As a result, the couple was able to feel much more allied in the readjustment period. Problem solving was facilitated by carefully breaking problems down into smaller, more manageable components that the patient could complete on his own. Rather than feeling overwhelmed and discouraged, he began to feel more confident and worthy because of his mastery of new situations, which led to an increasing sense of optimism. Clear recommendations to his employer allowed for at least temporary reassignment to a job that did not require such a high level of visual–perceptual function.

In addition to providing behavioral therapy skills and neuropsychological testing, psychologists often represent the member of the team who has had the most specific training in research methodology. We believe that the best clinical programs involve the interaction of clinical, research, and training components that inform and influence each other. As discussed in chapter 7, research involvement also provides an important mechanism for dealing with the stress of being a caregiver for patients with life-threatening illness. Further, with an increasing social pressure to evaluate the efficacy and efficiency of treatment modalities, it is important that one member of the team be able to contribute specific knowledge on the methodology involved in refining and pursuing specific clinical questions in the area of psychiatry and oncology.

Because of the high cost of psychiatric care and the limited number of psychiatrists in hospital settings, it is often the role of the psychologist to provide program development in the areas related to health psychology. As a result of evaluation and therapeutic expertise, the psychologist has a sense of program development related to the particular needs of the oncology population. The hands-on work of coordinating oncology services or coordinating research and clinical interventions gives a psychologist a specific expertise in the needs and programs that would be valuable to an oncology population. In many academic and small community hospitals, psychology has played a major role in the development of various programs related to pain control and desensitization, as well as in the implementation of necessary groups to provide mutual support for patients and their families. The psychologist also, with psychiatric consultation backup, can provide inservice training for the various other disciplines that are working with cancer patients, including physical therapy, respiratory therapy, nursing, social work, and nutrition. In many ways, a psychologist is in a unique position to develop and implement various multidisciplinary kinds of approaches to the family experiencing a serious life-threatening illness.

The Unique Contribution of the Social Worker

There has been growing interest in the integration of social work into medical programs (Wallace et al. in press). Such marriages are beginning to produce more social work professionals who are comfortable with the medical population, knowledgeable about a variety of medical disorders and their consequences, and appropriately trained in such areas as the psychological effect of medication and other biomedical dimensions of care necessary to an integrated understanding of the medical patient.

The social worker has been regarded in many settings as a key member of a multidisciplinary health care team. Such inclusion is strongly warranted by the extent of research that documents both the importance of social factors and the presentation of medical symptoms (Barsky 1979; Mechanic 1972; Rosen et al. 1972), and in the progression of an adaptation to medical illness (Mechanic 1980). Members of our psychiatric oncology team, including the social worker, are currently involved in a major project to assess the role of social support in the psychosocial adaptation of lung cancer patients and their families. The understanding of the problems of any patient with cancer cannot be divorced from an understanding of his/her social network and environment, vocational and financial context, and so on. It probably remains true that the social worker is the member of the mental health team who is most familiar with community resources and issues involving financial aspects of health care. However, this is not necessarily so, especially for social workers who view themselves primarily as psychotherapists. Still, working with individuals in the psychological adjustment to illness, or even with couples and families, is not unique to the social worker. It cannot even be claimed that a systems perspective—for example, a family perspective—is the unique contribution of social work inasmuch as many major family therapy programs are conducted by psychiatrists. Yet it is true that since the psychiatrist in the medical setting is often extensively involved with medical issues, the social worker, by virtue of a systems orientation, is often in a position to play a major role in this area, given proper training. It has been suggested that patients themselves are more resistant to social workers who have an exclusive focus on emotional and intrapsychic issues to the exclusion of social context and environmental concerns (Silver 1974; Mechanic 1978). We contend that in contrast to intrapsychic attention, active coping and mastery take attention away from bodily concerns and bolster confidence and self-esteem. Thus it should be emphasized that in many instances of psychological distress syndromes not reflective of obvious psychiatric illness, it is *particularly appropriate to assist patients in specifically defining external problems that are manageable, helping them to focus on active coping strategies that are relevant, and encouraging mastery of these problems.*

In addition to evaluation and management of social/interactional problems, the social worker who is knowledgeable about community resources can play a significant role in improving the situation of the patient and family. The coordination of home health care, for example, can provide an important hiatus for the stressed spouse of a cancer patient. Knowledge of rehabilitative resources can be an important means of providing the patient with input that improves the patient's sense of control and mastery over physical damage. Addressing the concerns that many patients have about paying their enormous medical bills, and assuring adequate support for their families while the patient is disabled and cannot work, is a significant contribution.

It is sometimes stated that discharge planning is the unique function of the social worker. It is true that many of the details involved in discharge planning, such as phoning to locate appropriate nursing home placements, are often assigned to a social worker. However, as invaluable and important as this contribution is to the overall care of the patient, the psychiatric social worker who is part of a mental health team has a unique task that goes beyond a technical facilitator. To understand this task, it is important to understand the difference between being a social advocate and a clinical advocate (Wallace et al. in press). The social advocate, who is represented by the more traditional role of the social worker, works on behalf of the patient to assure maximum access to resources requested by the patient or physician. The clinical advocate, however, does not merely carry out suggestions that may seem logical, but performs an independent assessment of the patient's overall function, psychological status, and interaction with other people to assure that whatever plans are made are clinically sensible. The following example shows the clear disjunction between plans that may seem to make sense on the surface but which are clinically not sensible when examined more closely. The nuances involved in discharge planning for patients include an interaction in a variety of psychological and social system issues. Because social workers are most readily identified by physicians as the resource finders, and because many referrals for concrete services turn out actually to involve underlying psychiatric or counseling issues (Wallace et al. in press; Stoeckle et al. 1966), the role of the social worker is to bring to patients the biopsychosocial clinical perspective to which the worker uniquely has access.

A 60-year-old, Irish-American woman's long-awaited retirement was darkened by a diagnosis of bone cancer. Her 66-year-old husband of 40 years, who had recently retired from pipe fitting, seemed overwhelmed by the diagnosis and insisted that his wife not agree to radiation therapy despite the physician's thoughtful and careful discussion of the illness and its treatment. The social worker was asked to help the couple arrange for some medical supplies. In meeting with the couple to discuss what resources and supplies were already available for home care, the social worker learned that their grown daughters typically played an important role as family problem solvers in times of stress. A family meeting, therefore, was arranged. In the subsequent contact, the elder, 43-year-old, married daughter voiced her concern that her father would find the prospective loss of his wife unbearable and return to drinking, from which he had abstained for many years. The other daughter, 31 years old and unmarried, had always remained closely involved in helping out her parents and providing caretaking, although she maintained her own apartment. She was visibly worried about both parents, remarked that she just could not move in with her father in the eventuality of her mother's death, and began to cry. Her sister ignored the tears and commented with impatience that her father would not be able to afford the gasoline for the daily 60-mile round trip to the hospital should their mother need to stay much longer. At this point, the father asked why the medications and supplies had to cost so much.

The family agreed to meet with the social worker over the next few days to discuss the problem of transportation, finances, and arrangements for helping out at home. The younger daughter was helped to define the boundaries of her involvement in such a way that she could maintain her own independence and still be a source of support to her father. The cost of the medication was deferred by having the prescriptions stamped, filled in the hospital pharmacy, and put on the bill for longer term payment. Other necessary medical equipment was found to be covered by Medical Assistance, which was made available to the family because of each spouse's low Social Security payments and the patient's now high medical bills.

Optimal provision of concrete/environmental services requires a role more complex than that of a "technician" who works simply by referring to a manual of community resources. Sometimes a request for concrete assistance serves as the entry point for a patient in significant psychological distress. A professional social worker, by utilizing a clinical data base, can recognize the real issue at hand and not be misled into providing some service that misses the mark for the patient's actual needs. The enhancement of adaptation to cancer requires a social worker whose clinical training provides such concrete services differentially; that is, in a manner best suited to the particular psychological makeup of the patient in the social network.

The Unique Contribution of the Nurse-Clinical Specialist

The nurse-clinical specialist in psychiatry is a registered nurse (R.N.) who has gone on to a master's degree in a specialized medical area (in this case, psychiatry).

In the past decade, the nurse-clinical specialist has begun to play an important role as a member of the psychiatry consultation-liaison team (Barton and Kelso 1971; Lewis and Levy 1982; Nelson and Schilke 1976). The nature of the hospital milieu often creates major stresses for the cancer patient, just as difficult patients create stress for a hospital unit. The nurse-clinical specialist in psychiatry appears to be the most knowledgeable member of the team about the complex daily realities of the hospital/ward milieu, including the nursing group in care of the patient. Patient care is often influenced strongly by events taking place among the nursing staff. For example, if a new head nurse is hired on a particular unit, the resulting disruption in the program may make nurses less able to provide continuous and consistent care, at least temporarily. Problems affecting the staff always have some fallout on the patient care (Stanton and Schwartz, 1954). The nurse-clinical specialist is in the best position to have access to such information and to be able to interact with the system in an appropriate corrective fashion. Correspondingly, certain patients are especially difficult for the nursing staff to take care of—including those who have a personality disorder that makes them excessively demanding or seductive, those who frustrate the staff as a result of unresponsive pain (see chapter 6), and those who are of the same sex, age, and socioeconomic level as the nurses providing the care and thus create special strain because of staff overidentification. In the management of such difficult patients, the liaison work provided by the nurse-clinician can be a critical factor in helping the other nurses to be more objective and to provide better care. No other member of the team can interact with this subsystem as well as the nurses in terms of their approach to patient assessment and management. Nurse-clinicians are in a unique position to monitor the implementation of therapy plans and the response to treatment, by virtue of their medical background and the fact that they are usually more involved on a daily basis with patient follow-up than are the psychiatrists. The nurse-clinician, for example, can monitor the effectiveness of a pain regimen with a high degree of awareness of the medical side effects and drug interactions. When such medical knowledge is combined with training in the psychological aspects of illness and the function of the health care system, the nurse-clinician can provide a powerful therapeutic presence, as the following case illustrates:

A 36-year-old married white male, father of three daughters, and employed as an Emergency Room technician, was referred by nursing staff to the nurse-clinical specialist in psychiatry for evaluation of depression. He had been diagnosed four years earlier with a glioma of the spine. He had experienced progressive disabilities, and at the time of the referral had total motor and sensory loss below the waist resulting in intermittent fecal incontinence, urinary retention, coordination deficits, and focal seizure activity in his upper extremities. He also experienced intermittent severe headaches as a result of extension of the tumor cells to his brain.

Initially, the nurses asked for help to manage his depression. It was soon evident, however, that the major problem for the staff resulted from their strong identification with this patient, who was a former hospital employee, was about the same age as many of the staff, and possessed many admirable personal qualities. Nursing staff complaints about this patient initially were, ''He's not even trying. Why isn't he out of his room more, and talking with other patients?'' By gently confronting the head nurse, who set the tone for his care, the nurse-clinician specialist helped the staff to recognize their unrealistic need to ''normalize'' this patient. The staff was helped to alter their expectations that the patient initiate all contact and also moved his room closer to the center of the nursing activity. Following this increased contact, his depressive symptoms greatly improved.

Pain control then emerged as a second management issue that the clinical specialist dealt with over time. The medical staff feared ''addicting'' the patient. Paradoxically, the patient's general optimistic personality style made it more difficult for the staff to justify increasing the analgesic dose since he was often able to put up a good front for the visiting physician though he silently suffered at other times. The nurse-clinical specialist was able to educate both the staff and patient about pharmacologic tolerance and the need for increased doses of longer acting analgesics on a regular schedule. The patient's wife was also encouraged to be his advocate concerning pain medications to help her feel like a meaningful participant in the treatment. Nursing staff was taught skills in monitoring his responses to analgesics and were able to make meaningful recommendations to medical staff. As a result of close monitoring of this system, the severe headaches were greatly relieved.

The patient's consistent denial of his progressive deterioration and his labile hospital course created additional strains for the staff and family. Increased immobility, pain, and seizure activity would often be interrupted by several days of remarkable recovery in comfort level, mental status, and social involvement. During such periods of recovery, the staff often became angered and complained that the patient treated them like servants and the hospital like a hotel. Repeated staff conferencing was necessary to help staff recognize how tiring their sustained involvement had become and their own needs to pull away. A more consistent nursing plan was formulated by those nurses who found it least difficult to remain involved with the difficult situation.

Overall, the psychiatric liaison nurse was able to intervene effectually on many levels because of the possession of medical-surgical experience in addition to psychiatric experience, the development of a good understanding of the nursing system operant in the hospital, and the maintenance of a high degree of visibility (Berarducci et al. 1979).

Conclusions

This chapter has stressed some of the unique contributions of various mental health disciplines, but in practice they often overlap to a considerable degree. In addition, the descriptions are somewhat idealized and presuppose adequate training, ongoing supervision, and team integration. Unfortunately, the integration of such professionals seems to be the exception rather than the rule.

All mental health professionals see themselves as ''psychotherapists'' to some degree, who feel they can be helpful to patients by talking to them or their families. However, the training and supervision of each member of the team are variable. It is currently very controversial as to whether any one discipline can lay claim to unique expertise in psychotherapy. We feel that any of the professionals can be competent psychotherapists given appropriate training and supervision. However, as described in chapters 4 and 6, it is quite difficult to decide whether apparently psychological problems (such as discouragement, irritability, or feelings of wanting to quit treatment) are secondary to some psychological problem or are a result of some medical impairment. It is the likelihood of overlooking such masquerading medical disorders, especially in patients with major medical illness, that is the major danger for the patient in a system that functions to a large extent within the unique limitations of each discipline as well as its unique contributions.

"Why do you have various disciplines participating in psychiatric consultation anyway? Don't they all do the same thing?" Our response to these questions is our contention that the professional roles are separable and that each provides a unique contribution within a complementary clinical team. Each member of our team is in a position to do an initial evaluation of a patient since we use a uniform data base that covers a broad range of medical and psychological data, which is then presented to the other team members with a psychiatrist present on a regular basis. Areas such as psychotherapy and sociotherapy that traditionally have been in contention among the various mental health professionals are assigned to the team members on the basis of background and training in the area rather than on the basis of profession alone. While the psychiatrist is in a unique position as a diagnostician, the provision of competent psychotherapy and sociotherapy is not the special domain of psychiatry. We have applied our model specifically to the area of psychiatric consultation to oncology patients, but we feel that it also is applicable to other consultation settings. This model, of course, implies definite training implications for each discipline. The intent of preparing staff to participate in the model is not to make nurses into psychiatrists or psychologists into social workers, but rather to create an understanding by each team member of the issues necessary in a comprehensive biopsychosocial approach to patient care. First and foremost, psychiatrists should be physicians and their training should emphasize a strong medical and neurologic component along with psychopharmacology. The psychiatrist must be comfortable with biologic, psychological, and social dimensions of patient care and functions optimally if there is no *a priori* bias to seeing problems as "organic" or "psychological" but instead an ability to integrate a number of viewpoints and mediate a variety of inputs. Psychology must continue to provide expertise in neuropsychological testing to assess those subtle cognitive and processing impairments that elude the standard neurological examination. Also, expertise in behavioral technologies is required. Social workers must learn more about the psychological consequences of medical illness, as well as medications and their side effects, in addition to providing a conceptual model of patient illness behavior in terms of the interaction of the personality and social network. Nurse-clinical specialists are of unique value as their background bridges medical, psychological, and social system issues and they can interact effectively with the nursing network responsible for the daily primary care of the patient.

References

ANGELL, M.: The quality of mercy. *N. Engl. J. Med.* 306 (1982): 98–99.

BARSKY, A. J.: Patients who amplify bodily sensations. *Ann. Intern. Med.* 91 (1979): 63–70.

BARTON, D., AND KELSO, M.: The nurse as a psychiatric consultation team member. *Psychiatr. Med.* 2 (1971): 108–115.

BERARDUCCI, M., BLANDFORD, K., AND GARANT, C. A.: The psychiatric liaison nurse in the general hospital. *Gen. Hosp. Psychiat.* 1 (1977): 1166–72.

BERGMAN, A. S., AND FRITZ, G. K.: Psychiatric and social work collaboration in a pediatric chronic illness hospital. *Soc. Work Health Care* 7 (1981): 45–55.

BERNSTEIN, I. L.: Learned task aversions in children receiving chemotherapy. *Science* 200 (1978): 1302–1303.

BLOOM, B., AND PARAD, H.: Interdisciplinary training and interdisciplinary functioning. *Am. J. Orthopsychiatry* 46 (1976): 4.

BLUMBERG, B. D., AND FLAHERTY, M.: Services available to persons with cancer. National and regional organizations. *JAMA* 244: 1715–1717, 1980.

BRODSKY, C. M.: Decision-making and role shifts as they affect the consultation interface. *Arch. Gen. Psychiatry* 23: 559–565, 1970.

BURCH, J., AND MEREDITH, J.: Nurses as the core of a psychiatric team. *Am. J. Nurs.* 74: 2037–2038, 1974.

BURISH, T. G., AND LYLES, J. N.: Effectiveness of relaxation training in reducing adverse reactions to cancer chemotherapy. *J. Behav. Med.* 4 (1981): 65–78.

CAPONE, M. A., WESTIE, K. S., CHITWOOD, J. S., FEIGENBAUM, D., AND GOOD, R. S.: Crisis intervention: A functional model for hospitalized cancer patients. *Am. J. Orthopsychiatry* 49 (1979): 598–607.

DEROGATIS, L. R., ET AL.: A survey of psychotropic drug prescriptions in an oncology population. *Cancer* 44 (1979): 1919–1929.

DEROGATIS, L. R., MORROW, G. R., FETTING, J., ET AL.: The prevalence of psychiatric disorders among cancer patients. *JAMA* 249 (1983): 751–757.

ELL, K., AND MORRISON, D. R.: Primary care. *Health Soc. Work* VI (1981) no. 4, supplement.

FOGEL, B. S., AND GOLDBERG, R. J.: Beyond liaison: A future role for psychiatry in medicine. (Unpublished manuscript.)

GOLDBERG, R. J.: Management of depression in the patient with advanced cancer. *JAMA* 246 (1981): 373–376.

HARVEY, R. F., JELLINEK, H. M., AND HABECK, R. V.: Cancer rehabilitation. An analysis of 36 program approaches. *JAMA* 247 (1982): 2127–2131.

HOSTEIN, S., AND SCHWAB, J.: A coordinated consultation program for nurses and psychiatrists. *JAMA* 194 (1965): 163–165.

KALTREIDER, N., MARTENS, W., MONTERRASA, S., AND SACHS, L.: The integration of psychosocial care in a general hospital: Development of an interdisciplinary consultation program. *Int. J. Psychiatr. Med.* 5 (1974): 125–134.

KORANYI, E. K.: Morbidity and rate of undiagnosed physical illnesses in a psychiatric clinic population. *Arch. Gen. Psychiatr.* 36 (1979): 414–419.

KLIGERMAN, M. J., AND MCKEGNEY, F. P.: Patterns of psychiatric consultation in two general hospitals. *Int. J. Psychiatr. Med.* 2 (1971): 126–132.

LEE, S.: Interdisciplinary teaming in primary care: A process of evolution and resolution. *Soc. Work Health Care* 5 (1980): 237–244.

LEVINE, P. M., SILBERFARB, P. M., AND LIPOWSKI, Z. J.: Mental disorders in cancer patients. A study of 100 psychiatric referrals. *Cancer* 42 (1978): 1385–1391.

LEWIS, A., LEVY, J. S.: *Psychiatric liaison nursing: The theory and clinical practice.* Reston, Va., 1982.

LEWIS, C. E., FEIN, R., AND MECHANIC, D.: *A right to health: The problem of access to primary medical care,* New York: Wiley-Interscience, 1976.

LIPOWSKI, Z. J.: Consultation-liaison psychiatry past failures and new opportunities. *Gen. Hosp. Psychiatry* 1 (1979): 3–10.

———: Review of consultation psychiatry and psychosomatic medicine: II. Clinical aspects. *Psychosom. Med.* 29 (1967): 201–224.

LURIE, A.: Social work in health care in the next ten years. *Soc. Work Health Care* 2 (4), 1977.

MCKEGNEY, F. P., BAILEY, L. R., AND YATES, J. W.: Prediction and management of pain in patients with advanced cancer. *Gen. Hosp. Psychiatry* 3 (1981): 95–101.

MECHANIC, D.: Social psychologic factors affecting the presentation of bodily complaints. *N. Engl. J. Med.* 286 (1972): 1132–1139.

———: *Students under stress: A study in the social psychology of adaptation.* Madison, University of Wisconsin Press, 1978.

————: The management of psychosocial problems in primary medical care: A potential role for social work. *J. Hum. Stress* 6 (1980): 16–21.

MELAMED, B. G., AND SIEGEL, L. J.: Psychological preparation for hospitalization. In *Behavioral medicine. Practical applications in health care.* New York: Springer, 1980.

MEYER, E., AND MENDELSON, M.: Psychiatric consultations with patients on medical and surgical wards: Patterns and processes. *Psychiatry* 24 (1961): 197–220.

NASON, F.: Team tension as a vital sign. *Gen. Hosp. Psychiatry* 3 (1981): 32–36.

NELSON, J., AND SCHILKE, D.: The evolution of psychiatric liaison nursing. *Perspect. Psychiatr. Care* 14 (1976): 61–65.

NESSE, R. M., CARLI, T., CURTIS, G. C., KLEINMAN, P. D.: Pretreatment nausea in cancer chemotherapy: A conditioned response? *Psychosom. Med.* 42 (1982): 33–36.

ROBINSON, L.: Psychiatric liaison nursing 1962–1982: A review and update of the literature. *Gen. Hosp. Psychiatr.* 4 (1982): 139–145.

ROSEN, B. M., LOCKE, B. Z., AND GOLDBERG, I. D.: Identification of emotional disturbances in patients seen in general medical clinics. *Hosp. Commun. Psychiatr.* 23 (1972): 364–370.

SCHWAB, J. J.: The psychiatric consultation: Problems with referral. *Dis. Nerv. Syst.* 32 (1971): 447–452.

SILVER, G.: *Family medical care: A design for health maintenance*, Cambridge, Mass.: Ballinger, 1974.

SLEPIAN, F. W.: Medical social work in primary care. *Prim. Care* 6 (1979), 3: 621–632.

SMALL, E. C., AND MITCHELL, G. W.: Practical aspects of full-time liaison psychiatry in gynecology. *J. Reprod. Med.* 22: 151–155, 1979.

SOBEL, J. J.: *Behavior therapy in termainal care. A humanistic approach.* Cambridge, Mass.: Ballinger, 1981.

SOBEL, W. K.: Behavioral treatment of depression in the dying patient. In H. J. Sobel (Ed.), *Behavior therapy in termainal care. A humanistic approach.* Cambridge, Mass.: Ballinger, 1981.

STANTON, A. H., AND SCHWARTZ, M. S.: *The mental hospital.* New York: Basic Books, 1954.

STEINBERG, H., TOREM, M., AND SARAVAY, S. M.: An analysis of physician resistance to psychiatric consultations. *Arch. Gen. Psychiatr.* 37 (1980): 1007–1012.

STOECKLE, J., SITTLER, R., AND DAVIDSON, G.: Social work in a medical clinic: The nature and course of referrals to the social worker. *Am. J. Pub. Health* 56 (1966): 1570–1579.

TURK, D. C., AND RENNERT, K.: Pain and the terminally ill cancer patient: A cognitive-social learning perspective. In H. J. Sobel (Ed.) *Behavior therapy in terminal care., A humanistic approach.* Cambridge, Mass.: Ballinger, 1981.

U.S. DEPARTMENT OF HEALTH AND HUMAN SERVICES: *Coping with cancer. A resource for the health professional.* Bethesda, Md. National Cancer Institute, 1980.

WALLACE, S. R., GOLDBERG, R. J., AND SLABY, A. E.: *Clinical social work in health care: New Biopsychosocial approaches.* New York: Praeger Press (in press).

WILLIAMS, P., AND CLARE, A.: Social workers in primary health care: The general practitioner's viewpoint. *J. Roy. Coll. Gen. Pract.* 29 (1979): 554–558.

WINSTEAD, D. K., GILMORE, M., DOLLAR, R., AND MILLER, E.: Hospice consultation team. A new multidisciplinary model. *Gen. Hosp. Psychiatr.* 3 (1980): 169–176.

CHAPTER 9

Information Disclosure and
Treatment Refusals—The
Clinical Dimensions of Potential
Ethical Dilemmas

WHILE PROBLEMS INVOLVING disclosure of information and refusal of treatment are not unique to oncology patients, they somehow seem more dramatic and have attracted much attention in this specialty. This may be so, in part, because of the assumption that learning that one has cancer will be so devastating. Further, unlike the patients in widely publicized cases involving termination of life support systems, cancer patients are often alert and competent spokespersons for their own wishes. Because of the prevalence of cancer and the prolonged course in many cases, there are a large number of potential problem areas that involve both these issues. In dealing with patients who refuse treatment or in deciding what information to provide patients during the course of the treatment, the oncology caregiver routinely faces situations that appear to be dilemmas. Should a patient be permitted to refuse treatment when the reasons for refusal are not clear? Is is right always to insist that a patient be informed, and can it ever be in the interest of the patient to know less? Notwithstanding the burgeoning literature devoted to the ethical dimensions of these areas (Beauchamp and Childress 1979; Jonsen et al. 1980; Reich 1978;

Walters 1981), the clinician must frequently make decisions without the benefit of conferences or time for extensive reflection. However, many times the apparent ethical dilemma involving these two areas is actually a misperception of the underlying problem (Lo and Jonsen 1980). The clinician can fall into the trap of thinking the decision is whether "to tell or not" or whether "to accept refusal or not." In fact, as this chapter demonstrates, many of the apparent dilemmas can be resolved by a clinical approach that engages the patient in a process that elicits underlying psychological or system problems in the course of treatment.

Disclosure of Information

If one brings up the topic of disclosure of information in a group of experienced clinicians, the response invariably is a variety of anecdotal reports of an apparently contradictory nature. Some claim that withholding information sometimes proves to be the humane approach; others will tell of patients whose insistence on knowing detailed information characterized them as a model of an intelligent courageous patient. Other problems are commonly presented: situations in which the patient seems to want to know less than the physician wants to tell; situations in which a family puts the physician in a bind by not wanting the patient to know the truth; situations in which patients behave as if they do not know what the physician feels was communicated. Some providers publicly uphold their paternalistic approach to disclosure, asserting that their professional duty is to provide only as much information as makes sense for a particular patient at a particular time. Others maintain that it is the patient's right to know as much as possible. This basic conflict between the obligation to inform and the obligation to protect can create an ongoing strain for the clinician. Decision making is further complicated by the prevailing context of social values that strongly influence the practice of individual clinicians and patients. Currently, the paternalistic style of medical practice is definitely being challenged by a more consumer-oriented and disclosure-oriented value system.

While the debate about disclosure is easily fueled and carried on, the actual determinants of clinical practice are difficult to analyze. Despite the documentable shift to physician attitude toward increased disclosure, what actually takes place in the office has not been adequately studied. There is probably a significant gap between espoused attitudes and actual behavior (Blanchard et al. 1982). Furthermore, the nuances of the communication process make this area a difficult web to untangle. The provider may communicate, either by tone of voice or nonverbal expression, a message other than what the words themselves state. Disclosure may be masked by the use of words that are too technical or by euphemisms. Information processing will be inadequate when it occurs in a highly emotionally charged setting. The provider often assumes that a single communication will suffice, and that once something has been said, the topic has been addressed. Finally, even well-intentioned advocates of complete disclosure must make decisions about what to select from a relatively unlimited pool of possible information. Disclosure is always selective, and therefore is dependent upon the provider. A listener may be distracted by pain, anxiety, or information overload. Some may be limited by intelligence, vocabulary, or cultural orientation from taking advantage of generally available materials. Some may be afraid to ask questions or to bother the physician by further inquiry. The patient's personality may affect the process: Some will require more details, others will be confused by them; some may prefer an impersonal, scientific approach while others need the personal touch. Finally, the patient, consciously or unconsciously, may deny the information and behave as if it had not been presented.

How is the thoughtful and intelligent clinician to proceed given the societal pressure to disclose, the professional value to protect, and the inherent limitations of the communication process itself? All theoretical arguments in this area finally come down to particular events with particular patients. Decisions are always being made for better or worse. In any single case, it may be impossible to predict the outcome of either telling something or of withholding it, but it is important to recognize the strengths and limitations of each option. Specifically, physicians should be aware both of the arguments that support and those that oppose paternalism, and of the clinical skills needed to carry out either policy—protection or disclosure. Supporters of full disclosure at all times should have an appreciation of the clinical impact on patients and of the clinical skills necessary to deal with this. Supporters of full disclosure must also recognize the limitations inherent in the communication process. Whatever position is maintained, the clinician must develop skills in communicating, listening, and understanding patients as individuals.

Changing Attitudes Toward Disclosure

Attitudes toward disclosure have changed significantly over the past three decades. In 1953, in response to a questionnaire survey of 442 Philadelphia physicians regarding the issue of disclosure of diagnosis, 69% of these physicians stated that they usually did not or never told their patients. Thirty-one percent said that they always or usually told the patients (Fitts and Ravdin 1953). In 1960, a survey of 5000 physicians found that the percentage stating that they never told the patient the diagnosis had dropped to 22%, while 16% of the group stated that they always told the patient (Rennick 1960). However, a broad change in social values influencing medical treatment by the early 1960s cannot be claimed; 90% of respondents to a survey of 219 physicians in Chicago in 1961 stated that they generally did not inform patients of their diagnosis (Oken 1961). By 1970, according to another, relatively small questionnaire survey, 25% of physicians always told the patient, and 9% never told the patient (Friedman 1970). A more thorough population survey was conducted by Novack et al. (1979) in Rochester, N. Y. In this study, which represented multiple specialists, 98% reported that it was generally policy to tell the patients. Two thirds stated that they never, or very rarely, made exceptions to that rule. These data are in sharp contrast to the earlier studies. The most frequent factors reported by physicians as intervening in their decision to tell the patient were the patient's age, the patient's intelligence, the patient's (and relatives') expressed wish about information, and perception of the patient's emotional stability. Yet how these factors actually related to the effects of imparting information about diagnosis remained largely unexplored and suggested that *a priori* personal judgments based on some attitudes and biases were the real determinants of policy. Eighteen percent of the sample reported they were less likely to tell a child and only 10% reported being inclined to tell an elderly patient or one who had poor comprehension. Fourteen percent said that they would tell the patient less frequently, or might delay telling, if they thought the patient was prone to depression or suicide.

Approximately 12% would tell the patient somewhat more frequently if personal business needed to be put in order. Hardy et al. (1980) more recently reported on a group of 185 physicians 97.7% of whom reported that they "always" or "usually" inform patients of the diagnosis. Factors reported to be important influences on decision making included: stage of disease (71%), age of physician (65%), treatment required (60%), family wishes (60%), histopathology (58%).

There are several possible interpretations that may account for the *attitudinal* changes reported in Novack's and Hardy's reviews of physicians' attitudes toward disclosure. Oken suggested, around 1960, that the diagnosis of cancer implied the expectation of death, depriving the patient of hope, and hence physicians were reluctant to tell cancer patients their diagnosis. (Paradoxically, 100% of the same sample indicated a preference for being told if they themselves had cancer.) Yet, by the late 1970s, physicians were telling the patients the diagnosis much more often. Part of this change perhaps could be accounted for by improved therapy that would allow physician to be more optimistic about their patients. Another factor that may have contributed to (or coincided with) the trend to increased disclosure has been the upsurge of interest in death and dying, with a consequent opening up of previously taboo topics. Finally, the swing in the pendulum of social values toward consumerism and increasing public scrutiny of the medical profession have altered the physician–patient relationship. Whichever factors are actually possible, it appears that oncology providers cannot escape the clinical issues that emerge as a consequence of carrying out the ethical demands of informing patients.

Problems in the Process of Disclosure

Few, if any, studies have considered exactly what or how physicians provide information to their patients in day-to-day practice. Despite evidence of changes in underlying attitudes, controversy over actual practice continues between proponents of guarding individual rights and their opponents, who claim that the attempt to achieve full disclosure is impossible because of limitations in patient understanding as well as the desires of patients not to want to be told (Meisel 1981). Do people want to know the "truth?" How can the clinician determine how much a particular patient wants to know? Can the "truth" be harmful? Are there any data available that can shed some light on these questions?

Meisel and Roth (1981) have reviewed the empirical studies in the area of informed consent, an area that has considerable overlap with the issue of disclosure. They found few, if any, studies that attempted to determine actual daily practice, though several studies have looked at some of the communication problems in this area (Golden and Johnston 1970; Boreham and Gibson 1978). Studies on whether patients want to be told appear contradictory. Some have found substantial numbers of patients who claim not to want to be informed (Alfidi 1975). In one study (Hinton 1980), more than 75% of the patients surveyed recognized that they were dying of cancer and communicated that knowledge to staff members who displayed an attitude of openness. These patients indicated they preferred frank communication with their caregivers and were happier when such openness prevailed. In a review of nine other studies in the area, Veatch (1978) found a significant majority of patients (60 to 98%) indicated the wish to be told a diagnosis of a terminal illness. Kelly and Friesen (1950) found that 98% of cancer patients indicated they preferred knowing their condition. However, McIntosh (1976) reported of the incurable patients he studied, almost half did not want confirmation of their diagnosis, none wanted to know whether the illness would be fatal. Henriques et al. (1980) studied a large sample of Danish patients with abdominal diseases, asking if they wanted to be told their diagnosis if it were cancer—54% said definitely yes; 22% probably yes; 8% probably not; 3% definitely not.

Unfortunately, there seem to be no studies that systematically examine whether disclosure causes "harm" to patients and what the nature of that harm might be. There has been some suggestion that informed consent can be "hazardous" to one's health (Loftus and Fries 1979), although there is also evidence that the benefits of information can be considerable (Brody 1980). Methodologically, studies of disclosure are quite difficult and would certainly need to involve real patients with serious conditions, rather than healthy subjects responding to hypothetical situations. Possible "negative consequences" would have to be carefully specified. Available studies on the negative consequences of disclosure have also been contradictory, with one demonstrating an increase in "apprehensiveness, anger, and anxiety" (Lankton et al. 1977), with another (about an impending surgical procedure) claiming to show a decrease in anxiety (Denney et al 1975). Cassem and Stewart (1975) cite studies indicating patients' overwhelming positive attitudes in favor of being told their diagnosis and a lack of demonstrable negative effects. Overall, there is a paucity of studies in this area and those currently available are of generally little help for the oncology provider.

Despite Novack's (1979) finding that 97% of physicians (in his sample) preferred to tell the patient their diagnosis, it is still not uncommon to find situations in which the patient behaves as if the physician had not done so, at least not in a way the patient has been able to process. For example, the physician may note in the record that "a full and frank discussion about diagnosis took place today," only to find that the patient continues to behave as if unaware of important elements. At times, this may be accounted for by low retention of information given to patients in stressful medical situations (Robinson and Merav 1976; Leonard et al. 1972; McCollum and Schwartz 1969, Reading 1981). Since patients may not recall much information when the timing of it coincides with peak emotional stress, one wonders whether disclosure can take place usefully in a single frank discussion, even when the clinician makes an effort to take into account the patient's intelligence, interest, and so forth. In some cases, patients are told things in a language that is too technical, or in euphemisms which obscure the situation. Furthermore, there are times when the diagnostic information is inherently uncertain and such a message may be translated by the patient as not being clear information, when actually there is no clear information to give. At times, the patient and family may collude in creating ambiguity to avoid confronting the reality of the diagnosis. The following case indicates the clinical complexities involved in attempts to provide information and some of the forces that determine how it processed:

> Mr. W., a 68-year-old, retired accountant, was diagnosed with prostatic carcinoma after almost a year of chronic weakness and fatigue. After getting pathologic confirmation of the diagnosis, the family physician, who had known the patient all his life, decided that this patient would be better off not knowing that he had cancer. The patient, for his part, gave repeated messages that he did not want to hear about having cancer. He said that he knew he had some chronic illness that was getting worse, but that learning he had cancer would certainly kill

him. While denying the reality of his diagnosis on one level, he nevertheless cooperated with all diagnostic and therapeutic measures without seeming to be bothered by the apparent paradox of receiving such extensive treatments for some illness he was convinced was not cancer. In this case, it was the patient's son who seemed more concerned about getting information. He was a highly educated, intelligent professional stockbroker for whom information was an important way of dealing with anxiety. Yet, despite his efforts to pin the doctor down as to exactly what was going on in treatment, he confided to a nurse involved in home care that he really did not understand whether his father actually had cancer or not. Despite having been given the pathology report to read, he claimed that the doctor was being evasive with him. It was possible that the physician was keeping things from the son as well as the father. However, an alternative explanation eventually emerged as a result of a careful clinical assessment. The son, himself, was ambivalent about getting decisive confirmation of his father's diagnosis and prognosis. As long as some ambiguity remained in the information, some hope remained that the illness was actually a benign chronic condition. The son held on to this possibility since the family physician originally had thought that was the case, despite confirmation to the contrary from oncology consultants later on. Just as the father coped by a fairly extreme form of denial, the son coped by a more moderate form. Part of his adaptation to his anxiety and need to "do something" was taken up by his search for more "information" from second and third opinions, which he used to contradict each other so he could keep the truth up in the air.

Disclosure of information is often not possible in a single or simple transmission event. It is a process that must take place over time and that requires a clinician who can analyze and comprehend a variety of psychological processes. Let us say that the physician accepts the premise that a single communication cannot, for many reasons, fulfill the intent of providing adequate information. This implies that the physician must continually monitor the "information status" of the patient and continually reinfuse information as the capacity of the patient changes in terms of anxiety, physical status, receptivity, etc. This process places an increasing burden on the provider who, as a consequence, must face the difficulty of repetitively informing. The difficulties of providing unpleasant, and often upsetting, news are multiplied. Further, the provider continually faces a dilemma of whether it is wise to "insist" that the patient be and act "informed." The provider may be in a position of having to challenge the patient's denial, and thus possibly undermine an important defense. It requires great skill to approach a patient who is maintaining denial. These dilemmas are highlighted in the following case:

> Mr. P. is a 52-year-old systems analyst who was "never sick a day in his life" until he consulted a physician because of excessive fatigue and difficulty in speaking. A positive brain scan led to the diagnosis of a brain tumor, confirmed on biopsy to be astrocytoma Grade III, located in the dominant hemisphere, parietal lobe. After several weeks in the hospital receiving radiation therapy, he began to complain of pain for which no medical explanation could be found; therefore, a psychiatric consultation was requested. The patient was found to be aphasic; he had great difficulty in expressing himself, often using incorrect words and remaining silent when asked questions. His affect was rather impassive. When asked why he was in the hospital, he said that he was having trouble with his arm and leg. Indeed the patient did have some weakness and numbness on the right side of his body. When asked if anything else were wrong, he said no. When asked to explain what sort of treatment he was getting, he would reply, vaguely, that he was getting treatment to make his arm better. When asked how he felt about his situation, he gave no clear response. To the suggestion that he might be feeling discouraged, he shook his head and indicated that he was not.

The oncologist had met with both the patient and the patient's wife several times to explain clearly that the patient had a serious brain tumor requiring radiation therapy. The wife understood what was involved in her husband's treatment. As for the patient, it was no longer clear what he understood about his situation. Apparently, people had tapered off talking to him about his diagnosis for a number of reasons. As long as he was participating willingly in his treatment, his denial of the brain tumor was considered by some as protecting him from being overwhelmed by his feelings. Denial was viewed as adaptive. There seemed little point in upsetting the patient by getting him to talk about a brain tumor that he clearly wanted to pretend, on one level, was not there. If his behavior were such that he was not participating in treatment, it would be necessary to confront the issue, but this was not the case.

Also, since that patient was seen as aphasic, it was not clear that discussing the situation with him would be very useful. In any case, it was extraordinarily difficult to sit with the patient and discuss anything because of his difficulty in speaking. Finally, given the location of the tumor in the part of the brain related to speech, some felt that the patient was neurologically impaired in terms of his ability to process what was going on and would only be confused by more information that he could not integrate. This case, therefore, raised a number of issues about ongoing communication of information. Certainly, if it was necessary to be sure the patient continued to understand what was going on, it was going to be necessary to "confront" the patient with things that had been gone over in detail previously, and to which the patient perhaps had adjusted in his own way. In a joint interview with the patient and his wife, the consultant (with the wife's prior permission) mentioned that the doctor had certainly discussed with both of them the presence of the brain tumor and that it was somewhat confusing as to why the patient appeared not to understand what was going on. The patient again said that his problem was with his arm and leg, that "they don't seem to work right," and he would not acknowledge the presence or effects of the brain tumor. It was then pointed out to the patient that he seemed to have a great difficulty in expressing himself. He acknowledged this. When it was suggested that he must have found this quite frustrating and perhaps was feeling cut off from his wife and family because of his speech difficulty, he became tearful and for the first time in the interview seemed "connected" with the discussion. He was told that we could understand how isolated he felt and that we would be sure to go slowly enough with him to make sure that he had the feeling of remaining in contact with us despite his speech difficulty. The patient (and his wife) seemed relieved at this. Plans were made for a social work therapist to spend time with the patient to help avoid the possibility of his isolation and to allow him the chance to express both feelings and questions about his situation. This case demonstrates that neither informing the patient nor the patient's awareness is an "all-or-none" phenomenon. In this case, the patient was able to acknowledge his speech deficit while he maintained the position of denial (for the time being) about the brain tumor. This has been referred to as "middle knowledge" by Weisman (1979) in reference to a situation in which the patient denies the condition but behaves as if he or she knows that it is present. The patient was not overwhelmed by mentioning the brain tumor. Useful information could be provided about the speech difficulty at this time in the patient's course. He was able to acknowledge a deficit related to it and was relieved that people could understand the problem. This case demonstrates that it is often necessary repeatedly to present information to a patient and not make assumptions about current or potential understanding.

How can a clinician handle a situation of working with a patient who apparently does not know the diagnosis? The clinician should not assume anything. Instead, through a series of questions, patients gradually should be led to reveal their experience of the illness, treatment process, and their level of awareness of what is going on. We have developed a semistructured interview (see the Appendix A), which, especially in the first section may offer some ideas for questions that facilitate the unfolding of information without excessive intrusion or anxiety. The patient is allowed to maintain denial if necessary, but is also invited to open up areas for more discussion. It is the obligation of the clinician to provide such an opportunity and to listen carefully to spot clues that the patient wants to continue. The clinician would contend that it is important *first* to understand the patient's experience before following through on any general intervention policy regarding methods or details of disclosure. The individual bias of the clinician must be supplemented as much as possible by the unique life data of the particular patient. For example: how has the person dealt with similar situations in the past? What is the family style of dealing with such situations?

Nurses often find themselves in the difficult situation of having to deal with patients who apparently do not know their diagnosis or do not have information about their current status or prognosis. The nurse who is involved in ongoing care, who feels restricted from disclosing information, faces an intolerably difficult situation. How can one work with a patient if basic information (e.g., about diagnosis) is excluded from discussion, especially when the patient seems to be wondering about it in some way? Avoiding the topic, changing the subject, or applying bland and vague statements can arouse feelings of deception and a sense of absurdity. In such situations, it is the general clinical sense that ''patients know anyway'' even if no one tells them directly. If so, the strain of maintaining a charade is even more telling.

The nurse whose inquiry leads to a discovery that the patient actually wants to know more, and is prepared to deal with it, faces additional dilemmas. By simply stepping in as the source of information, the nurse can run some risk of severing the patient–doctor relationship or creating a triangular relationship that may be difficult for the patient to manage. As an alternative, it may be useful to involve the patient in a discussion of what has made it so difficult to talk with the physician. Such a discussion may lead to ways to help the patient become a more effective self-advocate in his or her own treatment process. It is important not to deprive some patients of a sense of their own efficacy by taking away opportunities for self-initiated action. A knowledge of the patient's personality is important in making this decision (Goldberg 1983). It may be necessary psychologically to explore the patient's perception of the treatment system, or fears involved in not speaking up (for example, worry about taking up the physician's time, worry about being perceived as stupid, etc.). More cognitive structured approaches have been developed to help patients move from a passive stance to that of active participant (Sobel and Worden 1982) in these situations. If none of the strategies to get the patient to initiate ongoing discussion work, then the nurse must make a decision in which the ethics governing the nurse–patient relationship come into conflict with the ethics governing the nurse–doctor relationship (Yarling 1978).

The strain created by lack of information unnecessarily isolates patients and can create an atmosphere of mistrust and perplexing communication. The perceptions of children and old people are generally underestimated, and those groups are at special risk for not receiving appropriate information. The lack of information also may deprive patients of coming to terms with their own existence and paradoxically may increase stress through the torment of fantasies conjured up to fill the void.

Paternalism and Disclosure

Does an ethically informed policy of full disclosure help the clinician confronted by the patient with life-threatening illness who, in the midst of some routine care, looks up and asks, ''I'm going to make it, aren't I?'' Of course, there is no single answer that is correct each time this question is raised. The comforting pat on the shoulder may be just the thing needed; at other times, it could be grossly inappropriate. Only the clinician can attempt to decide what the question means. Is is a request for reassurance, a plea for companionship, a way for the patient to break out of isolation, a genuine request for information?

The clinical approach values action that is "in the patient's overall best interest." This position has been seen by some as excessively paternalistic. It has been pointed out that medical expertise is no guarantee of moral wisdom, and that the clinician's idea of the patient's "overall best interest" always involves some hidden evaluative component (Veatch 1972). Physicians begin from a position of paternalism. The heritage of the profession creates this stance. Physicians felt, and were probably right 50 years ago, that people would approach them as God-like figures and would say "Take care of me. I have pain in my back; tell me how to make it go away. I don't want to understand what's causing it. I don't want to understand that I have this or that option." Options were not offered. Even today, one hears physicians say, "People pay me to take care of them, not to educate them. I'm to do the worrying for them." Many people now disagree with this position.

One clinician recognized the dilemma he faces as a result of the power inherent in his role:

> A question I suffer and sweat over is wondering when my paternalistic stance toward patient care is persuading a patient because I have so much power. Who can stand up against me when I say, "Look, it would be a good thing to . . . ?" And what's involved in persuasion? I want to be sure I'm not brainwashing someone. I might be making what seems to be a better educated or healthier decision, but after all the patient is in a better position to see what he truly prefers.

Many arguments have been raised against the paternalistic position (Hoffmaster 1980). One of the most detailed critiques of this position (Buchanan 1978) has singled out several issues that might trouble the thoughtful clinician. For one, can the physician ever have sufficient knowledge to know what is really in the "best overall interest" of another person? If one argues that it is unlikely that one could ever know enough about a person to guarantee that a paternalistic approach is justified, then would not the same argument apply to the act of providing information as well as of withholding it? Underlying such debates, of course, is the question of whether the physician has some moral/professional obligation to play this role at all. If physicians become technicians and not healers, then it may be appropriate to abandon this role. Buchanan argues that no physician (or nurse) is in a position to make judgments about the quality of someone else's life. Hoffmaster (1980) points out the Catch-22 of such a stance:

> The nature of the issue precludes participation of the person whose life it is. When a physician has diagnosed a terminal illness and is debating about whether to inform the patient about it, he cannot ask the patient, "If it were discovered that you had terminal illness, would you want to know about it?" or "If it were discovered that you had a terminal illness, would you regard being informed about the terminal illness or not being informed about the terminal illness as leading to a more fitting completion in your life, when your life is viewed as a unified process of development?" Merely raising such a question would certainly be a tip-off to the patient about the severity of his disease. Thus the only person who, theoretically, is in a position to make such a judgment is, for practical reasons, excluded from making the judgment. Yet someone has to make the judgment.

What skills might be important for making such a decision and does the physician (or nurse) possess these skills? To begin with, paternalism requires a *pater*, a parent, someone who knows the patient in depth and detail. The physician's ignorance of the patient's values, culture, and life-style can be as detrimental to good care as the patient's ignorance of medical factors (Kleinman et al. 1978). It seems that a consultant or occasional contact is almost disqualified from paternalistic activity inasmuch as only the primary provider who has known the patient (and family) over time can make a claim for such knowledge. This is not to say that many specialists do not become involved with their patients to such an extent that they are not in a position to do the same. In-depth knowledge of the patient, then, seems a prerequisite for a paternalistic position. Such knowledge would require an ongoing relationship, exploration of the patient's subjective value, and knowledge of the patient's psychological resources. Even when the physician or nurse possesses the skills to elicit such information about a patient over time, how certainly can future responses be predicted? While the warnings to the paternalistic position are clearly sounded, there remain strong proponents of such behavior as a morally valued aspect of the physician's effectiveness (Cross and Churchill 1982) and of the fact that most patients, no matter how well informed, need the physician to choose for them at times (Ingelfinger 1980).

Conclusions

Physicians' attitudes toward disclosure have changed considerably over the past several decades. However, exactly what they say, how they actually say it, and the impact of such decisions have not been adequately addressed. Disclosure cannot take place in the form of a single "telegram." The process of assimilation of information must be recognized by the clinician who intends to provide information in an assimilable form. The assumption that there is a simple answer to the question of disclosure should be replaced by the intent to create an ongoing dialogue with the patient. Maintenance of such a dialogue challenges the clinician to develop skills such as how to identify psychological defenses, as well as are awareness of the clinician's own feelings, as for example, concerns about being the bearer of bad tidings.

The ethical principle that upholds the obligation to disclose information to the patient is currently in the ascendency. Perhaps this position is an appropriate corrective measure for excessive arbitrary witholding in the past. However, even when the clinician recognizes the need to have this ethical position guide behavior, informing the patient is a complex clinical process and not a simple matter of information transmission. The standards that guide medical behavior cannot displace the requirement for the provider to know the patient and understand the meaning of an event or a procedure for a particular patient (Katz 1978). Changing attitudes that lead to more disclosure must be accompanied by a recognition of the appropriate psychological and emotional support that a patient's knowledge may demand. The more that patients are told, the more they respond, either in words or by actions that require improved observational and listening skills on the part of both the physician (Saunders 1969) and nurse. It has been suggested that disclosure of information is analogous to giving a blood transfusion: "Like a transfusion of blood, the dispensing of certain information must be distinctly indicated, the amount given consonant with the needs of the recipient, and the type chosen with a view of avoiding unfavorable reactions" (Meyer 1968).

Refusal of Treatment

Mrs. M. is a 53-year-old, married woman whose diagnosis of renal carcinoma was made after she began to complain of pain in her arm. Never one to run to the doctor, she was finally convinced by her husband to see a physician, who made a diagnosis of a pathologic fracture of the humerus, secondary to tumor involvement. Referral to the oncology service led to further diagnostic testing, which revealed widely disseminated renal cell carcinoma. She was passively complaint with the diagnostic process, listened quietly to her physician's explanation of her disease, and asked few questions. She interrupted her silence finally by refusing the initial recommended treatment, which was pinning of her humeral fracture and radiation therapy. She insisted that there must be some medication that could heal her arm and said she would not come into the hospital or agree to surgery or radiation. She also indicated that she wanted no other form of treatment for the underlying cancer and became inaccessible to further discussion, continuing to insist that "muscle relaxers" were all she needed. Her husband and daughter seemed uncertain about what to do. At this point, members of the oncology service began to sense a dilemma: Should they be more persuasive or respect her decision, given the poor prognosis? Discussion about the case began to focus on how difficult it was to accept a patient's decision to refuse active treatment even though it might be ethically reasonable.

While a patient's refusal of treatment may raise an ethical dilemma for the clinicians involved, the question also must be asked: To what extent does a patient's decision reflect a rational choice that should be respected and when should the clinical evaluative powers of the clinician be brought to bear? Many, but not all, cases of refusal of treatment represent transition points in the ongoing process of the cancer experience for patients. These transition points may require a clinical management approach that is often overlooked. In the "old days," refusal of treatment was seen primarily as disagreement with the physician and was considered by some to be *prima facie* evidence of mental incompetence. After all, what rational person would not listen to the physician? Times have changed, but some element of this attitude lingers on. At times, psychiatrists may be called upon because of the feeling that something must be "wrong" with the patient to refuse treatment.

For patients, the appearance of the psychiatrist often confirms their sense that they are being viewed as wrong or incompetent for exercising autonomous judgment regarding treatment. Such perceptions can make it difficult to get close enough to talk to patients who, as a result of the disagreement and perceived insult, may have a hostile and protective attitude toward any more discussion of their decision. A stalemate is often reached in which the clinician becomes fixed on one recommended course while the patient becomes locked into another course of action. As already mentioned, sometimes the stalemate is maintained by the patient's resentment of the attitudes of the providers; at other times, it may reflect a defensive closing-off of any further pain that could be caused by having to reconsider a difficult decision. Sometimes an oppositional stance is the result of the patient's personality (Goldberg 1983). It may even be a symptom of an organic mental disorder or depression (see chapter 4). In still other cases, it may be a displacement of anger from some family problem or some nonspecific retaliation against a world perceived as unfair. Because there are so many possibilities, it seems important to engage the patient who refuses treatment in a discussion of the situation. One might ask, "Why make things worse by calling in a psychiatrist?" The best person to deal with refusal could be the oncologists themselves. However, for several reasons, this may not be so. Discussions in this context can be quite difficult for nonpsychiatric physicians since they require highly developed interpersonal skills and a sensitivity to psychological process. After all, the occasion for the contact is already highly changed by feelings on both sides. In addition, it might be too much to expect an unbiased investigation of the problem by the oncologist, not only because that role inherently may require too much of a sense of commitment to active treatment to be able to consider alternatives, but also because the oncologist automatically represents a biased "medical" position to the patient. It is unlikely that the oncologist could say, "It really doesn't matter to me which way you go with this; I'm here to help you think through what you want." You could even say it would be impossible for any oncologist to do that. Any physician, by virtue of the M.D. degree, may represent a biased position. It may be that the patient refusing treatment should meet with a nonmedical person, who is not identified with the treatment *per se*. To some extent, patient advocates are currently playing such a role in some oncology settings. In other settings, this role will be filled by a psychiatric consultant, or a member of that service. The psychiatrist who is familiar with the medical interface is in a good position to help sort out clinically the many factors that are potentially involved in refusal of treatment.

The initial moments of meeting with the patient are critical, and often decide whether the contact will be therapeutic. Our approach is represented by the dialogue that typically occurs with patients who refuse treatment, in this case with a patient who changed her mind about accepting chemotherapy after entering the hospital.

RG: What's your understanding of why I've been asked to see you?

PT: You're here to talk me into getting chemotherapy.

RG: Well, if that's what you think there's really no purpose in our going any further.

PT: What . . . ?

RG: Well, if you think I'm here to talk you into or out of anything, then it's really a waste of time for both of us.

PT: What do you mean?

RG: Well, I understand you're at a very important point in your illness now. Times like this can be very difficult. It often seems that things are happening at such a fast pace that you really don't feel as though you have a chance to think through everything as you might like to. It feels as though people are pressuring you.

PT: (nods)

RG: Well, I'm here simply to provide an opportunity for you to create some space—a time out—a chance to let things settle down a little and to talk about what's happening.

Of course, no approach at engagement always works, but this approach is generally successful in initially engaging most patients in this situation. There is no need to put off the patient with overly "psychiatric questions" such as, "What seems to be bothering you?" In fact, most patients can be encouraged to talk about their current situation by asking questions about the illness itself, such as those that are indicated in the first section of our semistructured interview (see Appendix A). The first section of this interview, especially, provides many insights into the private, subjective experiences of patients and much about their initial perceptions of their illness and treatment experiences that have formed the background for the situation they have reached in refusing treatment. Whatever issues are uncovered, they can often be addressed clinically by saying, "Whatever way you decide to participate in further treatment, it sounds as though there is a problem here that we should address." In the course of this review, a number of possible reasons leading to refusal of treatment may emerge that may be categorized as either *intrapsychic, interpersonal, systemic,* or *psychiatric.* It should be pointed out that in all of the brief vignettes provided, the patient's refusal of treatment seemed on one level to be a perfectly reasonable choice. Engaging the patient on the topic of the refusal decision might raise certain ethical questions that should be borne in mind, such as: Is the physician using persuasive powers to manipulate the patient into a decision that the patient actually would prefer not to make? From the vantage point of this chapter, patients who refuse treatment should be addressed by those who are trained to engage them in a process that attempts to take into account their unique needs. Treatment refusal often proves to represent an expression of some other underlying issue. However, one cannot escape the ethical dimension solely by redefining the problem in terms of clinical process, since the clinical approach often has a value bias hidden within it. Are not many of the decisions to refuse treatment actually options that some reasonable people (though not everyone) would choose? The frequency with which a clinical inquiry uncovers important, remediable concerns of the patient has reinforced our practice of a clinical, noncoercive approach. The following issues are always considered:

1. *Intrapsychic issues* that involve personal, psychological meanings that people attach to events. Such private, subjective views can lead to excessive anxiety, fear, or denial, and then to refusal of treatment. Such meanings may be "borrowed" from previous experiences of family or friends. What do the symptoms *mean* to the person? What does the treatment *mean* to the person? It is quite likely that someone else's experience will be "transferred" to the present. If the patient's uncle had been treated unsuccessfully for the "same" disease ten years before, the patient may feel there is no point in going through with the treatment now. Issues of whether the uncle indeed had the same disease or whether new treatments are now available may not become part of the patient's rational thinking process unless such items are explicitly uncov-

ered and corrected. Such borrowed distortions are so common that they should be routinely inquired about. One patient with a highly curable form of Hodgkin's disease was adamantly refusing treatment until it was uncovered that he thought his disease was the same as a highly invasive and malignant cancer that had led to radical head and neck surgery in one of his business associates.

Family "myths" in this area are especially powerful intrapsychic determinants of behavior. Anyone who has a medical condition that "runs in the family" can appreciate how difficult it is to be rational about that disorder. There is a powerful underlying feeling that somehow the same medical fate will overtake other family members. For this reason, it is important to obtain a family history as a way not merely of uncovering genetic risk factors, but also of uncovering "psychological risk" factors. If everyone were completely conscious of and comfortable with such material, all the clinician would have to do would be to ask: "Is there anyone in your family who has had a similar symptom or illness, and if so, what happened to that person, and are you concerned about that in a way that is affecting your current decision making?" In actual practice, no one would ask this question, and very few could answer it directly. However, such information can be crucial, and can be obtained more indirectly simply by taking a careful and unhurried family history which gives the patient the opportunity to say something about each first-degree relative. The interviewer must observe and listen carefully for indications of affective elements entering into the otherwise factual review. Whenever the patient talks about someone in a way that seems to reveal some unresolved feelings, the interviewer has a clue to inquire more about that person.

> One patient who was insisting on leaving the hospital rather than continue chemotherapy revealed in such an interview that her "favorite cousin" had recently died on the very floor of the hospital she was now on. This fact accounted for her feelings of wanting to get away and were successfully addressed (initially) simply by transferring floors (though the feelings were later addressed in more depth, allowing the patient to express some of her unexpressed and unresolved grief over the death of her cousin). Another patient, whose sudden refusal of further chemotherapy seemed incomprehensible, became very tearful in the review of family history when talking about her mother's death from a stroke ten years previously. Further inquiry into

the death revealed that the mother had been sitting watching T.V. with the patient when she suddenly grabbed her head, complained of a terrible headache, vomited, and passed out. The patient recalled some of her frantic feelings and the moment at the hospital when she was told her mother had died. She remembered that the doctors told her they had given her steroids, which were a component of the chemotherapy she was now refusing. Her own refusal of treatment somehow involved complex feelings of sadness over her mother's death that were reactivated, anger with the doctors for not saving her mother (which she was partially projecting onto her current physicians), and fears that steroids were a drug used only when death is imminent. Further discussion of these issues resulted in a calmer, more cooperative patient who was better able to participate in her own further treatment decisions.

2. *Interpersonal issues* consist of feelings emerging from current relationships with friends, family, or members of the treatment team. Some patients may reject their physician's recommendation because of mistrust. It is always important to find out about the patient's earlier experience with the medical system.

One lung cancer patient was refusing any radiation or chemotherapy and was about to leave the hospital when some important experiences with his treatment were uncovered during an interview. The patient was asked such questions as: What were the symptoms you first noticed that made you think that something was wrong? What did you think of doing about that? What did you finally do? Whom did you see and how did you choose that doctor? What happened on your initial visit? What were you told about your illness? By this point, the patient had revealed that he had symptoms of burning chest pain for over seven months. During that time, he had seen his physician four or five times and was always told that he had a hiatal hernia and that the burning pain was due to acid reflux. Finally, when the symptoms worsened and he insisted that more testing be done, a diagnosis of lung cancer was made. At this point in the interview, it was impossible to know whether that physician had indeed "missed the diagnosis" as the patient presumed, or whether he had two different medical problems, a hiatal hernia and lung cancer, which no physician, no matter how careful, could have diagnosed initially. In either case, the patient was angry with the physician and mistrustful of the treatment recommendation. The patient had secretly decided that he would leave the hospital and find someone else to treat him. In this case, bringing together the patient and physician to discuss the patient's perceptions led to a resolution of the patient's feelings and willingness to continue with his current treatment situation. The willingness of the physician to discuss the patient's feelings and acknowledge his perceptions was seen by the patient as evidence that the physician was trustworthy after all.

A further question that can elicit crucial data in the interpersonal domain is: "Who has been hit hardest by your illness?"

One woman with recurrent breast cancer was refusing to accept any further forms of active treatment. Her wish to arrange for admission to a hospice unit was accepted with some difficulty by her family and physician, perhaps because it seemed out of character with her action-oriented personality. However, her decision seemed to represent a viable option of refusing further active treatment, especially because the prognosis seemed relatively poor and the patient sounded so intelligent and rational about the decision. However, a single interview with the patient and her husband led to a different outcome. The purpose of the interview was not to change the patient's mind but simply to discuss her decision and to help the couple clarify its implications and some of the details involved in making further arrangements. During the interview, the patient became more withdrawn and upset, eventually apologizing tearfully to her husband for being such a burden. The theme of her concerns of excessively burdening her husband and those around her became more and more of an issue in the discussion, and eventually it appeared that while this woman may actually have opted for continued active treatment, she felt it would be unfair to her family and friends. After the opportunity to address this issue, of which her husband was not aware, the woman was able to arrive at a different decision about treatment. The husband reassured her about his support and told her the greater burden for him would result from knowing he had not been able to stand by her through whatever happened in her illness.

3. *Medical systems issues* emerge as a result of communication problems and discoordinated treatment in the complex world of medical care.

A 60-year-old lymphoma patient had just completed an exhaustive diagnostic assessment by hematology-oncology specialized treatment team in a large general hospital. He began to express his intention to leave the hospital and have no further treatment for his condition and his feeling that he was not sure that the diagnosis and prognosis were correct. In this case, the treatment team was very understanding and aware of some of the potential problems that had resulted in this outcome. The attending oncologist realized that, as with many cases, there were so many physicians involved in the diagnostic process that the patient had become confused and was reacting by pulling out of the system. Therefore, the attending sat with the patient, made clear that he alone would be responsible for the communication of medical information, and offered the patient the chance to ask questions. It seemed as though this intervention would be successful since the patient was very appreciative of the opportunity and acknowledged that the physician was correct in identifying problems that had occurred. However, the patient did not change his mind about leaving. A further interview with the social worker brought a new piece of information to light. The patient truly respected the attending oncologist in the hospital but simply felt that his long-time general practitioner, who was about 110 miles away, was really the only one from whom he could accept a medical recommendation. The patient said he was afraid to offend the oncologist by telling him about this and felt in a bind that could be resolved only by leaving the hospital.

A special three-way meeting of the patient, oncologist, and family practitioner led to mutual agreement about the treatment originally proposed.

The treatment involved for some stages and types of cancer can be so aggressive and invasive that many reasonable providers often wonder whether the cure is worse than the disease. When there is a judgment that the "odds" are in favor of the patient, most will encourage the patient to go through the rigors of treatment. However, when the situation is perceived to have uncertain or marginal gains, there may be significant ambivalence involved in enlisting the patient, despite the general tendency of physicians always to provide active treatment. When many providers are involved, including multiple physicians and nurses, the patient may be given conflicting signals about what it makes sense to do. These problems created by the clinicians are, of course, multiplied by the patient's own ambivalent concerns about participating in the treatment offered. The combination of patient and staff ambivalence can result in refusal of treatment. This can be a difficult problem to address. As a basic rule, one clinician should be in charge of coordinating communication from the medical team. However, even then the patient cannot be shielded from nonverbal attitudes expressed by other staff. The patient will be confused if the oncologist suggests one course of treatment, and there is a sentiment on the part of the floor nurses that the recommendation is inappropriate. At times, the consultant will have to arrange for a meeting of attending physician and nursing staff to discuss treatment and be to agree on a way to avoid catching the patient in the middle.

4. *Psychiatric issues* such as delirium, dementia, depression, or psychosis can lead to refusal of treatment. Cancer patients obviously can become confused because of metastatic consequences of the disease or brain metastases (see chapters 4, 5). In addition, significant and often remedial depression may result in changes in the patient's perceptions about treatment (Goldberg 1981).

In the course of the interview, it may be clarified that the refusing patient is actually in the midst of a profound depression or organic mental disorder that may be impairing judgment. There is no escaping the covert ethical bias inherent in medical care—the aim is to treat patients, to sustain life, and sometimes to do this at a cost that seems to violate certain other ethical imperatives for the patient's own autonomy. What do we do with a depressed patient who refuses therapy? Is this situation different from that of a nondepressed patient who refuses therapy? The unwarranted assumption—''Wouldn't you be depressed if you just relapsed with cancer?''—has been discussed in several earlier chapters, and it is hoped that the reader at this point can appreciate the need to address depressive symptoms from a biopsychosocial perspective with the hope of identifying a reversible component. It is our feeling that when there is any likelihood of recovery, every attempt should be made to evaluate and treat depression before accepting a patient's refusal in that context. In a sense, the depressed patient is considered incompetent during that state. Many patients in this situation grudgingly agree to treatment of their depression. Two weeks later, when in a nondepressed state of mind, they will reassess their decision to participate in further medical therapy, and even may say, ''I'm glad you didn't listen to me when I was that way; I was not myself.'' If the psychiatrist agreed to forego treatment of every depressed patient who professed lack of interest (the lack of interest and pessimism are themselves core symptoms of depression), many people would be deprived of restoration of their health. These are the kinds of quiet, everyday ethical dilemmas the clinician faces. The thoughtful clinician attempts to balance respect for the patient's choice (even when it might not seem the best choice to the medical value system) with the value that leads a physician to persuade the patient to go a little further in the hope of restoring the patient's capacity to think things through more clearly. Of course, the rationale for persuasion seems clearer when the depression seems likely to respond to treatment or can be identified as likely to be secondary to some correctable medical cause (as opposed to some degree of depressed affect involved with circumstances alone). The rationale to provide treatment is also clearer when an organic mental disorder is identified as a cause of impaired thinking processes. For example, hypercalcemia can cause temporary paranoia; excessive use of tranquillizing medication may cause attentional disturbance and impaired judgment, and so on. In such cases, these underlying discrete problems should be addressed, and the larger issue of refusal of other treatment considered when the patient is no longer delirious.

Sometimes the medical team looks to the psychiatrist to make a diagnosis of incompetence even without the presence of a diagnosable mental disorder as an excuse to force through some treatment decision they feel is in the patient's best interest. A recent article points out the dangers of using a psychiatric consultation to mask what is actually an underlying ethical dilemma (Perl and Shelp 1982). In one of their cases, a 70-year-old man with no previous psychiatric history was being treated surgically for metastatic osteosarcoma of the right hand. After several amputations had failed to arrest the disease, a further procedure was recommended in which the right arm would be disarticulated at the shoulder joint. The patient declined all further treatment and asked to be discharged home. A psychiatric consultation was called to evaluate "depression." It was apparent that the referring physician had sought the psychiatrist's help in persuading the patient to have additional surgery. At issue is what action was morally required given the circumstances of the case. In the assessment, the authors note that the patient was found to be "distressed" but his decision-making ability was not impaired. He and his family were offered counseling by the staff, but they declined further psychiatric contact. Other supportive services—pastoral care and social services—were made available. Eventually, the patient's wishes were respected, and he was discharged home. One of the issues, of course, lies in the phrases, "offered counseling" and "made available." So much depends on how these are done. As with the case of disclosure, the agreement to provide information does not specify the style of how it is offered. Similarly, the ability to engage a patient in a review of a decision depends to some extent on the agenda of the clinician and on the clinician's skills in engaging the patient. This realization, that a skilled clinician might be able to talk a patient into something that reflects the clinician's own bias, increases the ethical burden on the clinician. The corollary, that the attempt to engage the patient may fall short because of lack of clinical skills or a halfhearted attempt, increases the necessity to be aware of one's underlying ethical bias and also points to the importance of advanced interviewing skills. In addition, the psychiatrist must learn to recognize when the medical diagnostic framework is being misapplied and must know when to point out, "Look, you're using me inappropriately here. This is a competent, albeit depressed, person."

5. *Accepting Treatment Refusal:* As a final possibility, after appropriate reviews, the patient's wish to refuse treatment may be respected. In this instance, the clinician recognizes that the patient's choice represents an option in a world in which different people hold different values in terms of weighing and balancing issues such as survival versus quality of life. Whether or not one should participate in a treatment that might minimally prolong survival at a high cost in terms of quality of life is a matter of values. The nature of value questions is such that at base we should expect plurality of opinion. While rational discourse about options is important and possible, we must recognize and distinguish questions that are value dilemmas, on which in the long run we should not necessarily expect to come to agreement, from questions that are basically scientific, factual, or empirically determinable, and in which we should reach agreement if the discussion is rational. There can be a fine line between things that are just factual and psychological issues and those that are really value issues. Unless clinicians can learn to identify when a value dilemma is present, there is little possibility of dealing with it in an ethical manner.

An example of a value dilemma is represented by the opportunity, in late-stage cancer, to use an experimental drug. In such a study, sometimes known as "Phase II" study, there is an opportunity to try an experimental drug to see how it might make a tu-mor shrink, or how toxic it is, and there also is a slight chance of causing some remission of disease. Oncologists in a position to in-volve patients in such studies usually receive some benefit in terms of research from enrolling patients in these trials; however, since the oncologist is also the patient's clinician, there may be a conflict of interest. For the patient, it is often a quality-of-life decision. A patient offered a Phase II trial may have a 50/50 chance of dying in a month either way. With the drug, the patient might vomit a lot more, but there is also a 50/50 chance that with the drug the patient will have three good months before going through the month of dying. This seems to be a situation in which either alter-native is reasonable—to refuse such treatment or to accept it. This is the place where it is extremely important to recognize the value dilemma. Upon being offered this option for a child with cancer, it would be perfectly reasonable for a loving, well-meaning, and wise parent to say either yes or no at that point. But the physician who does not accept a plurality of values can bias the decision in either direction. The physician who does not like unnecessary suf-fering, does not like to cause a child to vomit who is going to die in a month, can say, "There's nothing available that will cure your son. Don't shop around. Let's concentrate on making him as comfortable as possible." Or the physician can bias the phrasing differently by saying, "Without this drug, he'll die. With it, he'll probably die, but at times there have been, albeit rarely, some prolonged remissions. Maybe something else will come along. I can't give you much hope of that, but it's all we've got."

The matter of phrasing is subtle and difficult to study since it requires actually hearing what physicians say and how they say it rather than accepting reports of their attitudes toward disclosure. Some parents will be sophisticated enough to analyze the phrasing and ask, "Exactly what kind of chances are you talking about? Has this ever happened to anyone else?" But most people will go along with the sense of what the physician recommends. Many people, regardless of demographics or clinical status, believe in the importance of such clinical investigations and approve of the altru-istic rationale that sometimes underlies their implementation. On the other hand, a sizable group disapproves of having patients serve as research subjects and does not attribute much significance to altruistic motivations (Cassileth et al. 1982). When the patient refuses further treatment, the physician faces a critical juncture. Physician behavior at this point can be either a positive or a negative force in keeping the patient under overall medical care. It is important to have discussed the pros and cons in a rational way and to accept the patient's decision without a punitive or angry undertone. "It is particularly important to reassure the patient that even as he or she chooses a treatment that the physician disapproves of, the patient may return at any time without prejudice for treatment" (Holland 1982).

Conclusions

1. Literature on the patient who refuses treatment and leaves the hospital "against medical advice" (AMA) reveals some consistent features. It seems that such patients are mainly influenced by factors occurring either at the time of admission or early in the course of hospitalization (Fabrick et al. 1968; Scheer and Barton 1974; Struen and Solberg 1970). This suggests that such behavior, rather than reflecting a breakdown in the therapeutic relationship, often reflects a breakdown or disagreement in the contracting process that takes place early in the course of treatment. Disagreement about the nature of the "treatment contract" has been identified as a variable that is of some value in predicting those patients who eventually will sign out of the hospital AMA (Steinglass et al. 1980). Another study of patients who left the hospital AMA found that there were three basic reasons behind the threat to leave: overwhelming fear, anger, and severe psychiatric reactions, including depression (Albert and Kornfeld 1973). The patient's expression of intent to break off treatment, in such cases, is the action of someone for whom no other solution seems available. Many patients prefer to resolve such a crisis if given the opportunity. When confronted with such a patient, the clinician should ask, "What in this hospital situation, including my own behavior, has provoked the turmoil this patient is now experiencing?" The patient's behavior should not be taken personally (Koumans 1965). Acknowledgement of real shortcomings of the system may be necessary; questions that have been evaded or greeted indifferently may need to be answered honestly. The openness demonstrated by taking a serious interest in trying to un-

derstand what is going on, in itself, goes a long way toward resolving some of the common systems issues of concern to these patients.

2. Refusal of treatment may be the outcome of some temporary alteration in mental status as a result of depression or some organic mental disorder, which requires diagnosis and treatment. When the derangement has been appropriately identified and corrected, the patient may be in a position to reconsider the question at hand.

3. Refusal of treatment may be the outcome of some psychological issue that has been raised by a problem in the treatment system, or may be a product of the patient's own intrapsychic process. This point is amply documented in the literature regarding patients who leave treatment against medical advice.

4. The consultative use of a psychiatry oncology team (see chapter 8) may be important in addressing the dilemmas raised by patients who refuse treatment.

5. Accepting the patient's refusal of treatment may be ethically justified in situations that a group of reasonable people would handle in a pluralistic manner. Recognizing and managing these situations requires that clinicians be aware of their own biases, as well as continued development of both the ethical and clinical perspectives. Inadequate clinical skills may lead to a decision that is as morally unacceptable as that arising out of excessive persuasion.

References

Albert, H. D., and Kornfeld, D. S.: The threat to sign out against medical advice. *Ann. Intern. Med.* 79 (1973): 888–891.

Alfidi, R. J.: Controversy, alternatives, and decisions in complying with the legal doctrine of informed consent. *Radiology* 114 (1975): 231–234.

Beauchamp, T. L., and Childress, J. F.: *Principles of biomedical ethics.* New York: Oxford University Press, 1979.

Blanchard, C. G., Ruckdeschel, J. C., Blanchard, E. G., Arena, J., Saunders, N., and Malloy, D.: Do attitudes predict behavior: Correlation of oncologist' attitudes with their observed behavior toward cancer patients. AACE Abstracts, 16th Annual Meeting, 49A, Nov. 1982.

BOREHAM, P., AND GIBSON, D.: The informative process in private medical consultations: A preliminary investigation. *Soc. Sci. Med.* 12 (1978): 409–416.

BRODY, D.: The patient's role in clinical decision-making. *Ann. Intern. Med.* 93 (1980): 718–722.

BUCHANAN, A.: Medical paternalism. *Philos. Pub. Affairs* 7 (1978): 370–391.

CASSEM, N. H., AND STEWART, R. S.: Management and care of the dying patient. *Int. J. Psychiatr. Med.* 1 (1970): 295–305.

CASSILETH, B. R., LUSK, E. J., MILLER, D. S., AND HURWITZ, S.: Attitudes toward clinical trials among patients and the public. *JAMA* 248 (Aug. 1982): 968–970.

CROSS, A. W., AND CHURCHILL, L. R.: Ethical and cultural dimensions of informed consent. *Ann. Intern. Med.* 96 (1982): 110–113.

DENNEY, M. D., WILLIAMSON, D., AND PENN, R.: Informed consent— emotional responses of patients. *Postgrad. Med.* 60 (1975): 205–209.

FABRICK, A. L., RUFFIN, W. C., AND DENMAN, S. D.: Characteristics of patients discharged against medical advice. *Ment. Hyg.* 52 (1968): 124–128.

FITTZ, W. T., AND RAVDIN, I. S.: What Philadelphia physicians tell patients with cancer. *JAMA* 153 (1953): 901–904.

FRIEDMAN, H. S.: Physician management of dying patients: An exploration. *Psychiatry Med.* 1 (1970): 295–305.

GOLDBERG, R. J.: Management of depression in the patient with advanced cancer. *JAMA:* 246 (1981) 4: 373–376.

————: Personality disorders. In H. Leigh (Ed.), *Psychiatry in primary care medicine.* Menlo Park, N. J.: Addison-Wesley, 1983.

GOLDEN, J. S., AND JOHNSTON, G. D.: Problems of distortion in doctor–patient communications. *Psychiatr. Med.* 1 (1970): 127–149.

HARDY, R. E., GREEN, D. R., JORDAN, H. W., AND HARDY, G.: Communicating between cancer patients and physicians. *South Med. J.* 73 (1980) 6: 755–757.

HENRIQUES, B., STADIL F., AND BADEN, H.: Patient information about cancer. *Acta. Chir. Scand.* 146 (1980): 309–311.

HINTON, J.: When do dying patients tell? *Br. Med. J.* 281 (1980): 1328–1330.

HOFFMASTER, B.: Physicians, patients and paternalism. *Man Med.* 5 (1980): 189–202.

HOLLAND, J. C.: Why patients seek unproven cancer remedies: A psychological perspective. *CA-A Cancer J. Clin.* 32 (Jan.–Feb. 1982): 10–14.

INGELFINGER, F. J.: Arrogance. *N. Engl. J. Med.* 303 (Dec. 1980): 1507–1511.

JONSON, A. R., CASSEL, C., LO, B., AND PERKINS, H.: The ethics of medicine: An annotated bibliography of recent literature. *Ann. Intern. Med.* 92 (1980): 136–141.

KATZ, J.: Informed consent in the therapeutic relationship: Legal and ethical aspects. In W. Reich (Ed.), *Encyclopedia of bioethics* volume 2. New York: Free Press, 1978.

KELLY, W. D., FRIESEN, S. R.: Do cancer patients want to be told? *Surgery* 27 (1950), 6: 822–826.

KLEINMAN, A., ET AL.: Culture, illness and care: Clinical lessons from anthropological and cross-culture research. *Ann. Intern. Med.* 88 (1978): 251–258.

KOUMANS, A. J. R.: Psychiatric consultation in an I.C.U. *JAMA* 194 (1965): 636–637.

LANKTON, J. W., BACHELDER, B. M., AND OMINSKY, A. J.: Emotional responses to detailed risk disclosure for anesthesia: A prospective, randomized study. *Anestesiology* 46 (1977): 294–296.

LEONARD, C. O., CHASE, G. A., AND CHILDS, B.: Genetic counseling: A consumer's view. *N. Engl. J. Med.* 287 (1972): 433–439.

LO, B., AND JONSEN, A. R.: Ethical decisions in the care of a patient terminally ill with metastatic cancer. *Ann. Intern. Med.* 92: 107–111, Jan, 1980.

LOFTUS, E. F., AND FRIES, J. F.: Informed consent may be hazardous to health. *Science* 204 (Apr. 1979), 4388: 11.

McCOLLUM, A. T., AND SCHWARTZ, A. H.: Pediatric research hospitalization: Its meaning to parents. *Pediatr. Res.* 3 (1969): 199–204.

McINTOSH, J.: Patients' awareness and desire for information about diagnosed but undisclosed malignant disease. *Lancet* 2 (Aug. 1976): 300–303.

MEISEL, A.: The exceptions to informed consent. *Conn. Med.* 45 (1981): 27–32.

MEISEL, A., AND ROTH, L. H.: What we do and do not know about informed consent. *JAMA* 246 (Nov. 1981), 21: 2473–2477.

MEYER, B. C.: Truth and the physician. In E. Fuller Torrey (Ed.), *Ethical issues in medicine: The role of the physician in today's society.* New York: Little, Brown, 1968, pp. 166–177.

NOVACK, D. H., PLUMER, R., SMITH, R. L., OCHITILL, H., MORROW, G. R., AND BENNETT, J. M.: Changes in physicians' attitudes toward telling the cancer patient. *JAMA* 241 (1969): 879–900.

OKEN, D.: What to tell cancer patients: A study of medical attitudes. *JAMA* 175 (1961): 1120–1128.

PERL, M., AND SHELP, E. E.: Sounding board: Psychiatric consultation masking moral dilemmas in medicine. *N. Engl. J. Med.* 307 (Sept. 1981): 618–621.

PERLIN, S., AND BEAUCHAMP, T. L. (EDS.): *Ethical issues in death and dying.* Englewood Cliffs, N.J.: Prentice-Hall, 1978.

READING, A. D.: Psychological preparation for surgery: Patient recall of information. *J. Psychosom. Res.* 25 (1981): 57–62.

REICH, W. T. (ED.): *Encyclopedia of bioethics.* New York: Free Press, 1978.

RENNICK, D. (ED.): What should physicians tell cancer patients? *N. Med. Mat.* 2 (1960): 41–53.

ROBINSON, G., AND MERAV, A.: Informed consent: Recall by patients tested postoperatively. *Ann. Thorac. Surg.* 22 (1976): 209–212.

SAUNDERS, C.: The moment of truth: Care of the dying person. In L. Pearson (Ed.): *Death and dying.* Cleveland: Case Western Reserve University Press, 1969, pp. 49–78.

SCHEER, N., AND BARTON, G. M.: A comparison of patients discharged against medical advice with a matched control group. *Am. J. Psychiatry* 131 (1974): 1217–122.

SOBEL, H. J., AND WORDEN, J. W.: *Practitioner's manual: Helping cancer patients cope.* BMA Audio Cassettes, 1982.

STEINGLASS, P., GRANTHAM, C. E., AND HERTZMAN, M.: Predicting which patients will be discharged against medical advice: A pilot study. *Am. J. Psychiatr.* 136 (1980): 1385–1389.

STRUEN, M. R., AND SOLBERG, K. D.: Maximum hospital benefits versus against medical advice. *Arch. Gen. Psychiatry* 22 (1970): 351–365.

VEATCH, R. M.: Models for ethical medicine in a revolutionary age. *Hastings Center Report* 2 (1972), no. 3: 5–7.

VEATCH, R. M.: Truth-telling, I: Attitudes. In W. T. Reich (Ed.), *Encyclopedia of bioethics.* New York: Free Press, 1978.

WALTERS, L. (ED.): *Bibliography of bioethics.*, volume 7. New York: Free Press, 1981.

WEISMAN, A. D.: *Coping with cancer.* New York: McGraw-Hill, 1979.

YARLING, R. R.: Ethical analysis of a nursing problem: The scope of nursing practice in disclosing the truth to terminal patients. Part II *Supervisor Nurse* (June 1978): 22–35.

APPENDIX A

Semistructured Interviews for Patient and Spouse

STUDY #:___ GROUP #:___ INTERVIEWER: _____ DATE: ___

SEMISTRUCTURED INTERVIEW FOR THE PATIENT
(Coded Scoring Sheet Available from Author)

SECTION I. Prediagnostic Profile

1. How did you first become aware of your illness?
2. What made you finally decide to see a doctor?
3. Was there anything that made you hesitate about seeking help?
4. How did your spouse respond to your hesitation?
5. Was your spouse involved in getting you to seek help?
6. If your spouse was an important influence in arranging for medical evaluation, how much time was involved before he/she insisted on your getting help?
7. What were your own ideas of what caused those symptoms before a diagnosis was made?

SECTION II.

1. How did you hear about your diagnosis?
2. What did the doctor tell you about the illness?
3. What did you feel when you heard the diagnosis?
4. When people receive upsetting news, they often find certain thoughts going through their minds over and over again. What recurring thoughts have you experienced?
5. How do you feel your spouse has reacted to the diagnosis?
6. Who in your family has been hardest hit by this?
7. Did you and your family meet together with the physician to discuss your illness?
8. Was everyone in your family made aware of the diagnosis, or has there been a decision not to tell some people or to tell only parts to some people?

SECTION III.

1. How do you feel you will do with this illness?
2. What do you see for yourself in the future?
3. Have you discussed your illness with your employer?
4. Have there been any negative reactions at work?

SECTION IV.

1. What has been the biggest problem since your diagnosis?
2. How much have financial concerns been a problem?
3. How much would you say your relationships with friends have been affected since learning of your illness?
4. What have you told your friends about why you were (are) in the hospital?
5. How much pain have you felt as a result of your illness?
6. Have any family or close friends gone through a similar illness?

SECTION V.

1. Have you ever been treated for a nervous condition?
2. Has anyone in your family?
3. Habits: alcohol; tranquilizers; other drugs or medication?

SECTION VI.

Family Tree

(Include information regarding dates, causes, impact; also other people especially close almost like ''family.'')

SECTION VII.

1. Do you see yourself as a religious person?
2. How do you practice your religion?
3. Has there been a change since your diagnosis?
4. Have you spoken to clergy?
5. Do you believe in life after death?
6. In what way?
7. Prior to your present illness, what has been the biggest crisis you have had to face?
8. What got you through that?

SECTION VIII.

1. Are there any other issues that you feel it is important to bring up or for us to know about?
2. In addition to treatment at Rhode Island Hospital, have you thought about seeking other kinds of treatment?
3. How much help do you anticipate needing?
4. What kinds of services have you thought would be most helpful?
5. How has it been to discuss these issues?

STUDY #:___ GROUP #:___ INTERVIEWER: _____ DATE: ___

SEMISTRUCTURED INTERVIEW FOR SKO

SECTION I. Prediagnostic Profile

1. How did you first become aware of your spouse's illness?
2. What made him/her finally decide to see a doctor?
3. Was there anything that made your spouse hesitate about seeking help?
4. How did you respond to his/her hesitation?
5. Were you involved in getting him/her to seek help?
6. If you were an important influence in arranging for medical evaluation, how much time was involved before you insisted on his/her getting help?
7. What were your own ideas of what caused those symptoms before a diagnosis was made?

SECTION II.

1. How did you hear about your spouse's diagnosis?
2. What did the doctor tell you about the illness?
3. What did you feel when you heard the diagnosis?
4. When people receive upsetting news, they often find certain thoughts going through their minds over and over again. What recurring thoughts have you experienced?
5. How do you feel your spouse has reacted to the diagnosis?
6. Who in your family has been hardest hit by this?
7. Did you and your family meet together with the physician to discuss your spouse's illness?
8. Was everyone in your family made aware of the diagnosis, or has there been a decision not to tell some people or to tell only parts to some people?

SECTION III.

1. How do you feel your spouse will do with this illness?
2. What do you see for yourself in the future?
3. Has your spouse discussed his/her illness with his/her employer?
4. Have there been any negative reactions at work?

Copyright© 1982 by Richard J. Goldberg, M.D.

260

SECTION IV.

1. What has been the biggest problem since your spouse's diagnosis?
2. How much have financial concerns been a problem?
3. How much would you say your relationships with friends have been affected since learning of your spouse's illness?
4. What have you told your friends about why your spouse was (is) in the hospital?
5. How much pain has your spouse felt as a result of his/her illness?

SECTION V.

1. Have you ever been treated for a nervous condition?
2. Has anyone in your family?
3. Habits: alcohol; tranquilizers; other drugs or medication?

SECTION VI.

Family Tree

(Include information regarding dates, causes, impact; also other people especially close almost like ''family.'')

SECTION VII.

1. Do you see yourself as a religious person?
2. How do you practice your religion?
3. Has there been a change since your spouse's diagnosis?
4. Have you spoken to clergy?
5. Do you believe in life after death?
6. In what way?
7. Prior to your spouse's present illness, what has been the biggest crisis you have had to face?
8. What got you through that?

SECTION VIII.

1. Are there any other issues that you feel it is important to bring up or for us to know about?
2. In addition to treatment at Rhode Island Hospital, have you or your spouse thought about seeking other kinds of treatment?
3. How much help do you anticipate needing?
4. What kinds of services have you thought would be most helpful?
5. How has it been to discuss these issues?

APPENDIX B

Psychosocial Data Base

RHODE ISLAND HOSPITAL
DEPARTMENT OF PSYCHIATRY
PSYCHIATRIC CONSULTATION

(Page 1 of 3 pages)

NAME _____ | UNIT # _____

ADDRESS _____ | PHONE: _____

BIRTH DATE _____ S.S.# _____ | # YEARS SCHOOL: _____

REFERRED BY _____ REFERRAL PROBLEM: _____

PRIMARY CLINICIAN _____ OCCUPATION: _____ | B   W   H   ORIENTAL
RACE: AMER. INDIAN   OTHER

INSURANCE STATUS _____ SEX: F   M | RELIGION: J   P   RC   OTHER: _____

MARITAL STATUS: _____ S M D W SEP. | NO. OF CHILDREN: _____ | OCCUPATION OF PARENT IF SINGLE
OR SPOUSE IF MARRIED: _____

RESPONSIBLE PERSON: _____ RELATIONSHIP TO PATIENT: _____

ADDRESS: _____ PHONE: _____

VITAL SIGNS: BP _____ | PULSE _____ | TEMPERATURE _____ | RR _____

PATIENT'S CHIEF COMPLAINT: _____

HISTORY OF PRESENT ILLNESS: _____ INFORMANT: _____

_____

_____

_____

_____

_____

_____

_____

_____

_____

_____

_____

_____

SIGNIFICANT RECENT LIFE EVENTS: _____

_____

M-309 CAT. #2984771 REV. 6/81   **1**

RHODE ISLAND HOSPITAL
DEPARTMENT OF PSYCHIATRY

(Page 2 of 3 pages)

PAST PSYCHIATRIC HISTORY:

_____

_____

_____

_____

DEVELOPMENTAL AND SOCIAL HISTORY:

Perinatal Complications: _____ Infancy: _____

Problems Starting School: _____ MBD: _____

Anti-Social Behavior: _____

Other: _____

Living Arrangements: _____

Social Support: _____

Daily Activity: _____

Self-Care: _____

School, Work, Military History: _____

_____

HABITS (Alcohol, Drugs, Tobacco, Caffeine): _____

_____

FAMILY HISTORY (Psychiatric and Medical Disorders: Note Special or Stressful Relationships):

CURRENT MEDICATIONS (Dose, Duration, Recently Discontinued): _____

_____

_____

_____

MEDICAL HISTORY:

Allergies:	Surgery:
Head Injuries:	When Next Period is Expected:
Chronic Medical Problems:	Active Medical Problems:

M-309 CAT. #2984771 REV. 6/81 **2**

RHODE ISLAND HOSPITAL
DEPARTMENT OF PSYCHIATRY

(Page 3 of 3 pages)

PERTINENT NEUROLOGIC AND MEDICAL FINDINGS: _____

_____

_____

MENTAL STATUS EXAMINATION: Appearance: _____ Participation: _____

Organic Mental Disorder:		Psychotic Disorder:
Judgement:		Hallucinations:
Orientation:		Delusions:
Intellect:		Paranoia:
Memory:		Incoherence:
Affect:		Phobias:
Aphasia Screen:		Anxiety/Panic:
Affective Disorder:		
Mood:		Suicidal:
Sleep Change:		
Appetite:	Fatigue:	Homicidal:
Guilt:	Anhedonia:	
Psychomotor Change:		Personality:

DIFFERENTIAL DIAGNOSTIC IMPRESSIONS: Circle and Provide DSM III code if Confirmed:

_____

_____

_____

_____

DISPOSITION AND TREATMENT PLAN: _____

☐ Social Work   ☐ Behavioral Medicine

☐ Psychology Testing   ☐ Psychiatry

☐ Medical-Neurology-Surgery   ☐ Outside Referral

☐ Other Records

_____

_____

_____

_____

SIGNATURE: _____   DATE: _____

M-309 CAT. #2984771 REV. 6/81   **3**

Index